2 Corinthians 4:17

For our light affliction, which is but for a moment, worketh for us a far more exceeding and eternal weight of glory.

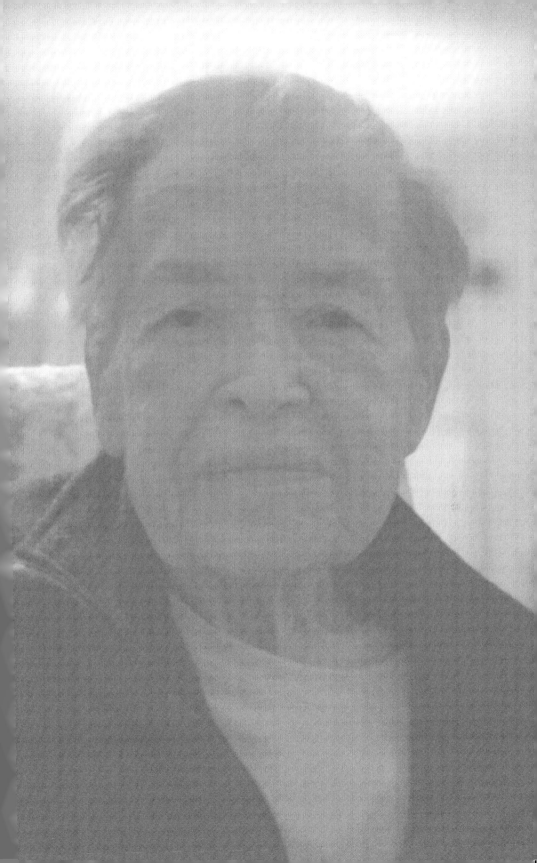

🌢

and just like that,

my tears became like rain

This is a personal journey of faith while traveling through one of life's most dreaded disease called Alzheimer's. If you are offended by the practice of Christian faith, then please tell me where you find your unfailing hope in the journey between life and death.

Table of Contents

    I.   Unpredictable Weather Patterns
    II.   Tracking the Storm
    III.   Anchored in Faith
    IV.   Dynamics
    V.   Submerged in Who They Become
    VI.   Beauty Within
    VII.   Steady Course

Lamentations 3:21-23

This I recall to my mind, therefore have I hope. It is of the Lord's mercies that we are not consumed, because His compassions fail not. They are new every morning:

Great is Thy faithfulness.

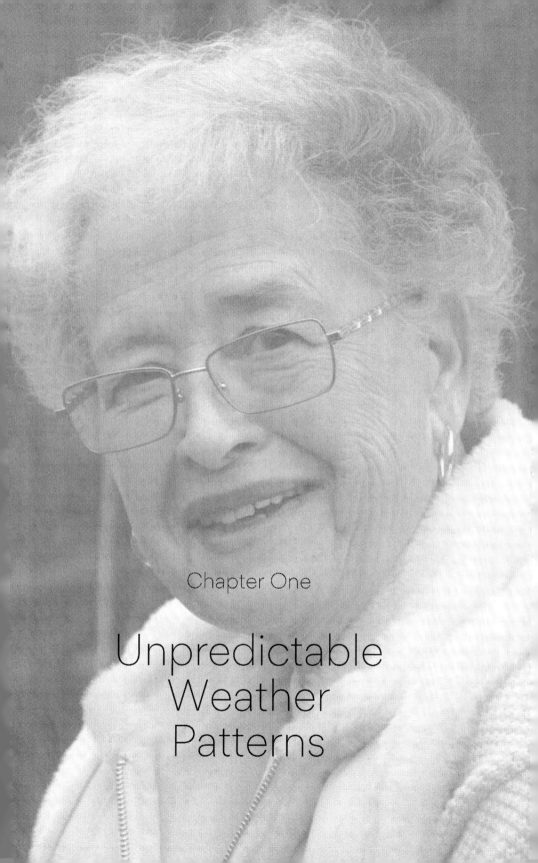

Chapter One

Unpredictable Weather Patterns

I could still hear thunder in the distance, yet the storm had already passed. Meteorologists track a storms' path so we can be prepared. Major storms are named and leave a path of destruction as if to show off its trail of devastation. Every storm is different. Weather patterns are unpredictable.

Amid our world, it was beautiful with a few spotty clouds but off in a distance, thunder was heard. I had already pulled down my patio umbrella. I had lost three umbrellas because of other storms. The sky soon filled with electrical charge. The clouds rolled by while trails of thunder and lightning appeared like fireworks across the sky. The wind blew but we did not get one drop of rain. I watched the red, yellow, and green images move across the screen of my weather tracker app. I was prepared for the storm.

But nothing had prepared me for the storm we experienced in mom's later years.

Mom hated storms, but in her last few years she became totally unphased by its passing. She didn't jump at the sharp claps of thunder anymore to shout "oh!" In fact, the remaining personality trait that even sounded like "her" was a sneeze and those were few and far between. Winds picked up speed and blew in all direction that swept through mom's character and personality like none other. She was eventually carried away with the tide by one of the most dreadful storms of all.

Alzheimer's.

The patterns of Alzheimer's are equally unpredictable, and I believe that everyone is affected differently. I am speaking both on behalf of the person and the immediate people surrounding them. Similar to scientific meteorologists, physicians track their path and learn from the different behaviors. Much is unexplained and like the weather; every day is different; every patient is different; every family is different.

May I interject here that my writings be received as an encouragement to you with whatever storm you're facing. It is purely written with that intention. Certainly not to press you with what you can expect from Alzheimer's effects but rather share from my perspective and how my family have personally weathered this storm. Medical research continues and I encourage you to stay connected with the physicians for possible treatments and direction. Above all, I wish you clear skies with hope in where you can place your permanent anchor. In the One who created the entire universe:

El Shaddai. God Almighty.

Looking back, I always wanted to become a nurse but was not able to pursue the education.

> I now realize that God called me to an honorary nursing position. That is to care for my mom.

I believe it is important to give proper introduction to her and the family that we represent. I know most would say not to be "friends" with your parents. But, sparing a few times during the awkward teenage years, my mom has always been my best friend this side of heaven. There has never been a time that I could not tell her anything that pressed my mind. Many times, conversations were tough though such as the dislikes of school or not having a boyfriend. Not feeling very pretty. With buck teeth, knot knees and bushy eyebrows it was no wonder I didn't have a boyfriend! I was not very popular. Wanting to do "what everyone else was doing" with her reply being "if they all jumped off a bridge…"

Being the daughter of a minister of music, we had strong standards to uphold.

                         Especially with the last name of HOOKER!

These Hookers were at church every time the doors were opened. We attended every funeral and in fact, we were good friends with the owners of the local funeral home. We attended most weddings because we were likely participating in them. When we weren't in the choir and were seen chatting too much in the congregation, mom would glare at us from the choir loft and we knew that was enough. If she were beside us during church and we were too loud, she would pinch the dickens out of our arm. It was crazy getting ready to leave our house for church on Sunday mornings. Someone would be playing the piano singing loudly, another would be on the telephone, a radio would be playing in the kitchen, another would be singing a different song in the bathroom and then there was me: watching TV and waiting until the last minute to get dressed only to change clothes twelve times before we left. "good Lord Donna," someone would say. I thought for years I was royal to be addressed as such.

We certainly all sang. Whether we had the talent or not, we all sang. Or at least, we thought we could sing because who does the choir director use when others won't do the special music? That's right. Family. We never really questioned it. We would get tickled at song phrases…"now let us…" and in our simplistic humor think that was SO funny as if we were saying "now lettuce…" Things are always funnier in church for some reason and our pew would shake from us trying to hold back the laughter at the least little thing. Someone always requested us to sing an unrehearsed song. Well, we were never really rehearsed with anything and in the words of my dad, we learned early to "just roll with it" and above all, smile.

Mom spoke fondly of her own younger years and loved to remanence about many stories of her family. Like the time they had baby ducks and she and her sisters eagerly watched them from the creekbank. They constantly shuffled them back into the water until the ducks were exhausted from swimming.

> Yet, the water was insignificant to those little girls.

She said the little ducks kept trying to swim ashore, but she and her sisters couldn't resist watching them in the water. Ducks are supposed to swim right? They have those little webbed rubber feet and the water rolls off their backs like beads. They soon noticed the ducks had become so tired they couldn't hold their heads up. The girls remedy? Wrap them in a towel and place them into their warm oven to dry off. Not to worry, somehow, they survived and mamaw didn't realize how close they came to having duck stew that evening. Even more and thankfully, papaw never found out. That storm would have been fierce.

Mom and her sisters were always close and loved to laugh together. A wonderful family heritage! Four sisters: Alice, *my mom was the oldest*, Lee, Clellene, and Betty. Those that spoke the loudest, had the floor. We loved to travel to visit mom's family in Pigeon Forge especially in the winter with the snow. Once, dad had to park our car at the bottom of the hill because we couldn't get our station wagon up the mountain. There were certainly no cell phones then. Every step we took, we slid three steps backwards while carrying our belongings. Well, if you call one large red suitcase family luggage, that contained our belongings and I guess my brothers took turns hauling it behind us. We were a sight. Papaw most likely watched us through his telescope and chuckled at us all. It was all we had but we were happy and couldn't wait to get there. It was a steep hike in the snow and at least we had our shoes and coats because it was about half a mile uphill (yes, the old cliché of walking to school uphill in the snow both ways). It was a special time in our lives. Over the years, we continued to stay very close with mom's family even though miles and life responsibilities interfered.

Mom was very artistic and loved to draw with charcoal and pencil. She devoted much of her time to drawing roses and her artwork revealed great detail. She loved working with her hands. She could knit, crochet, and sew.

All of her work was professional. She became a seamstress in her early career but as we grew older, she took interest with cosmetology. She loved her new direction and had the personality and talent that it required. She was a natural with people. She was eventually encouraged to advance because of her creative teaching abilities. She furthered her responsibilities and became a licensed instructor for most of her career and then retired as a State Instructor.

She was an extremely talented lady.

Being active in church and the community was important to her. She had many friends and people would call her often because she was a good listener. I never heard her complain about others. She would not consider herself strong, but she was. She loved humor and always made others feel better about themselves in any situation. We never went anywhere but what we ran into one of her friends.

When I was a young teen-ager, I listened to her talk to someone on the telephone one evening. Being confined to the length that the phone cord would allow during those days, she stood in the kitchen and shared words of encouragement. She hung up the receiver and said, "Donna, come with me to visit someone right now." Dialing emergency assistance did not exist at that time (other than dialing the operator) so without consideration of anything other than her friend, we drove across town. Her friend was in despair. Mom was fearful she would take her own life. I remember exactly where we were that night when we paid her friend a visit to talk. Mom never judged her but just listened and with confidence, prayed with her before we left. We weren't there long but long enough that it mattered to that lonely soul. I never knew the real story. I didn't need to know but I saw in Whom my mom trusted above all.

Jesus.

In the early 80's, our family withstood an unexpected loss. Our dad suffered a massive heart attack and was gone in an instant. The morning our dad died, he had a brief conversation with my oldest brother Sammy who ended by saying, "have a good day dad…" Dad's reply was "the best day of my life!" I didn't know about

Sammy's conversation until a short time ago when he shared it with me, but dad passed in 1982. It's something you never really get over, rather you learn to move forward every day. Since learning about that short conversation between a father and son at work, it has been a band aid of a reminder of my dad. Even though it crushed our world, it really *was* the best day of his life. Losing dad left a scar so deep in my heart that it has taken a lifetime for me to absorb. I vividly remember standing with my brothers during those visitation hours greeting loved ones with confident smiles in knowing where our father was.

In the presence of God.

For those left behind, trusting the Lord is the only comfort in dealing through the loss of a loved one and if by chance you are reading this, please be confident in knowing where your eternity will be. Don't gamble away another day. Just call on His name.

Jesus.

After the loss of dad, mom was suddenly forced to pick up and move forward. She didn't want to though.

> She battled some depression but eventually became more active with new things in her life.

She had to learn in the years to follow how to truly depend upon the Lord. She had a wonderful support around her with family and friends and day by day grew stronger. The Lord used her struggles as a lighthouse to others during their own trials.

Years later and what seemingly passed by quicker than anyone could blink, love led her to the alter with a wonderful gentleman named Bill. We grew to love Bill and he genuinely loved our mom which was the only thing that we cared about. They had approached around 10 years of marriage, and then another unexpected storm swept through our family while taking Bill with cancer.

I think the first time I truly saw mom exhausted was during the weeks prior to losing Bill. I was compelled to leave work because I didn't want her to be alone during those last moments and that time was fast approaching. She opened the door and almost fell into my arms. For once in my life, I was so thankful to have followed my heart with that visit. Within three more days, Bill was called home to heaven.

We had then approached a new phase in life that brought us back together with overnight visits. It was during those quiet evenings that I heard her first whispers of prayer. I don't think she knew her voice carried because she kept her voice soft like she was keeping secrets from others in a conversation. I couldn't even make out the words she was saying but Someone heard.

Jesus.

Before mom made the decision to move in with me, there were many episodes that I witnessed her do. After the loss of Bill, I visited her every Saturday and would sometimes follow her back from the local restaurant where we met up with other family members for breakfast. Driving home behind her one Saturday morning,

> …she turned up the oncoming lane instead of her own traffic lane.

I gasped because there was absolutely nothing I could do at that point but watch from behind. Thankfully, she corrected herself in time. During another driving episode, she sideswiped a neighbor's mailbox. She barely made it out of the shallow ditch and stopped her car. It did not do damage to the mailbox but left a nice long scratch on her car. Over time, she "turned in her keys." Sammy began picking her up for church and other events that she wanted to attend.

Navigation Check Point: Safety

- *Driving. Let's face it: as we age, our reflex is just not as quick or accurate. We can't stop as quickly if someone pulls out in front of us in traffic. It's not only dangerous for your loved one but for anyone within their perimeter. Now is a good time to enter conversations respectfully with them and discuss a plan during this transition. It's difficult for them to give up their independence but it is a necessary conversation to have. I recommend having a spare set of car keys made for yourself at this time since they repeatedly misplace items.*
- *Awareness. I watched mom become too trusting in public. She would plop her wallet onto any counter and get into a conversation while not paying attention to her surroundings. Anyone could quickly brush against her and be gone in a flash with her belongings. Become familiar with their outings and routines while they are still mobile and doing independent errands.*
- *Medicine. If they do not have someone to disperse their medicine on a routine basis, they can easily make fatal mistakes with their own medications. Make certain they do not stray from the physician's orders regarding prescription medicine. Become familiar with the pharmacist and certainly their primary care physician. They are a personal team of security for protection.*

We encountered a few times that mom would be out on short errands and get easily turned around. One particular time, she became turned around and looked for landmarks to help her determine exactly where she was but had to eventually call my sister-in-law (Debbie) for help. Deb told her to stay where she was at that moment, and she would come to get her.

As we approach our senior years, we begin to lose our way and may easily become disoriented in public or in traffic. What were previously familiar landmarks are suddenly gone when construction sites for renovations move in. This can present a very troubling course for seniors. Business names and locations frequently change in today's market but can easily alter someone else's direction. Most everyone today has a smart phone and for us at that time, it became increasingly difficult to find the type of phone that mom could operate. She was not able to remember phone numbers, but we kept immediate numbers in her contacts that she knew how to access, and she at least did a good job with keeping her phone charged. For those going through a similar transition, there are constantly new device options for seniors today that include cell phones, trackers, security cameras, location apps and more. It just takes the support people surrounding them so they can continue to feel independent and safe.

Understandably for our family, safety became a major issue. She was too trusting in public. Mom would carelessly leave her wallet open on any counter easily accessible for others to grab and be gone. Let alone the danger in her being hurt with any incident as such. We were also very concerned about her being out somewhere alone with risk that her blood sugar might quickly drop since she was a diabetic.

Mom also became very careless about her medications. Since she was a diabetic, she did a good job most of the time with controlling her blood sugar through her diet, but she was still prescribed routine medications. On a few occasions, she would become weak and during those episodes was fortunate to be with other family members for quick assist. Her pulse rate would fluctuate on occasion so with these health concerns at her age, we took extra care and frequently checked on her throughout the day.

Then like most storms develop and appear out of nowhere, unpredictable weather quickly moved in. There are many aspects to consider when you find yourself at a crossroad decision if you question dementia "symptoms" with someone.

> In the beginning of dementias, the person may recognize something is different but there is no expected time scale here. They are also clever in disguising their own concerns.

You can't think in terms of "this phase is expected to last three months." Note that forgetfulness may not be dementia at all but rather common absent mindedness with age. There are specific tests for dementia so please follow up with a team of specialists for a proper diagnosis and plan of care.

They are worried but don't want to express alarm. They want help but also want to seem normal. This begins a very confusing time for them. They want to keep their independence but need the security of someone close by. They begin repeating the same sentence multiple times and sometimes back-to-back in a simple conversation. They identify with photos in their younger years but may not recognize themselves. They begin to hide things (such as car keys) with a sense of paranoia so no one else will find the item. You can tell them as many times as you want to "keep your keys on top of the table" but they will inevitably tuck them into a drawer, purse, pocket or any odd little place so they (get this) won't lose them. They may develop an odd fetish such as collecting tissues. Mom always kept tissues with her but with the advancement of dementia, she would pull all tissues out of the box, refold them and tuck them into her pockets or purse. Many times, I would only find tissues in her purse stuffed to the brim.

You find yourself searching for logic to their odd behaviors.

It's much like taking the letters of the alphabet and tossing them into the wind. How many words can we create with the English alphabet? Yes, that's as many different behaviors and patterns that can appear. There is just no logic to it because we are all created differently, and our fingerprints and DNA are proof of that. We are all as different and as unpredictable as the weather!

Along this emotional chapter of my life, I found an outlet with writing. I openly shared on social media platforms about our personal journey. Mostly to encourage others that are entering this same storm. I mentioned many in our family that assisted mom through different situations. Many might think that someone within your own family that has a lot of "extra time" and would be able to "take care of" your loved one. Don't place that burden on someone unless they feel called to step in and help. There are many markers along this path and in most cases, once an action takes place, there is no turning back. The person becomes quickly dependent on the aid (whether that action is providing a ride for them to get groceries, assisting them with personal hygiene, doing their laundry or even staying together at overnight visits).

My writings are also shared candidly with regard to faith and is written in nonchronological narrative. I'm pretty certain that I have permission from my heavenly Father to quote Him at His Word too, but you can research His Word for yourself. That's what He wants us to do anyway. In case you wonder, I personally read and study King James Version which is the version that I reference in this journal.

> **Public Media Post**
> February 12, 2019
>
> I know from the prospective of Alzheimer's, there is fear. Vision is distorted. Hearing is still present but they are listening for the familiar sounds that comfort them. Music provides peace. Touch is very comforting. Holding their hand brings amazing security for them, and equally for us because we are searching for comfort too. Typically, when you think of fear you think of whatever stands between you and your safety but even more fearful...is the unknown.
>
> It's like staring into the vast ocean surrounded by water and depth. You wonder what is there. You feel the toss of the waves. You tighten your grip.

> There is no anchor. The waves begin to carry you further out of sight. You can't even determine the horizon because it fades into the sky. The wind carries you about and you have utterly no control of your direction.
>
> All navigation is lost.
>
> It's the same for Alzheimer's. Place yourself into the unknown world for just 10 seconds. What if you didn't comprehend anything except for the split second by split second. What if you weren't able to even put a spoon to your mouth or even verbalize that you were hungry? Because that's their reality.
>
> That depth in the ocean? That's the same lost stare coming from their mind.
>
> Mom still has good days though. This week, she has done very well but it's a false sense of well. We are extremely thankful that all through this journey, she is in a "happy" place. Hospice is a wonderful extended family. They cater to her and offer comfort to us. There is absolutely no timeline with any of it. There is no logic to any behavior or reaction which is so difficult to grasp. Questions we ask ourselves are the same questions professionals ask.
>
> Again, navigation is lost.
>
> We have simply chartered this course for the unknown but, at least we are sailing there together. And we will take every split second there is.

At the swell of the tide when your family must decide about caregiver needs in your own situations, be aware these are major decisions that will essentially place your social life and your personal life on hold indefinitely. It will bring about a ripple effect with everything. There are countless doctor visits. Your own well-being will be affected. Our family has been most blessed in that we are tightly knit together and demographically close in proximity. I understand that may not be the case with others. You may be a single child forced to make the decision demands with a parent or close member that has been diagnosed with a dementia. You may not have a choice at all. Or, perhaps you have siblings, but you all live in different states, or you may live within the same town, but your family is rather disconnected. It could just be that your own life responsibilities do not allow the added time to assist.

I do know that until you are faced with a major decision as such, you never know how you will really react. It's best to get as much professional advice and personal discussions with everyone involved to be accountable and on the same page but above all, begin with asking the Lord for help.

> Believe it or not, the simple prayer, "help me Lord!" is a literal miracle within itself…

…no matter how big or small your need. He will be there for you in ways you could never dream. His grace is amazing and endless.

Do you sense some unpredictable weather patterns forming?

I know in whom you can trust to navigate you through the storm.

Jesus.

Hebrews 6:19

Which hope we have as an anchor of the soul, both sure and stedfast.

Chapter Two

Tracking the Storm

Growing up in the 70's, I would go with my dad on "visitation" where he would spend his spare time and visit with people from church, work and the community. Sometimes, we would go to the nursing home and visit people there. Oh yes, and you bet we would sing! Those little people would roll into the "Activities Room" and be elbow to elbow lined up. They would call out to us and chatter constantly. They would grab us as we walked by. They had crumbs in their mouths while talking. Most didn't even have their teeth. They wore bibs. And there was this very distinct odor. We didn't pay attention at all with fear to the exposure of germs. We had a heck of an immune system growing up! It doesn't sound very pleasant, but we loved on them, and they LOVED in return. It made an impact on my life at a young age. I didn't understand or even question why they were there. They were just old and maybe didn't have anyone to care for them.

> I felt sorry for most of them and chuckled at their odd little behaviors.

Who would have thought these events would prepare me for what lie ahead in my own life.

I remember many times hearing mom and dad refer to someone having "hardening of the arteries" and I thought how terrible that would be. I questioned did our veins just harden with age? Would we begin to freeze in our movements? What did that mean exactly?

I didn't want to grow old.

I had never heard anything about Alzheimer's until the era of the 90's. I thought it was odd to occasionally hear on the news that an elderly person had been found roaming outside by themselves, lost and only wearing their pajamas…. or worse yet, barely clothed. I began to hear increasingly more that adults were reported missing by their family members. Many times, I would hear of those missing from nursing homes too. How could that happen? What were they thinking being outside at night with no shoes on their feet? Did they not realize how dangerous that was for them?

It reminded me of an unfortunate fellow in our hometown that would sit on the front steps of the Post Office. He was crippled and blind. He sat on the side of the steps with a cigar box for contributions of tossed coins from people as they passed by. He was there every day.

And there was another local fellow that roamed the streets with a big ball of string. He would carry it in his hands and while he walked, the string would trail behind him. I watched from the back seat of our car traveling to church, barely peering over the car door as we drove by. What on earth was that about? I never knew what these people suffered from. They could have been as content as ever, but it seemed they had fallen victim to circumstance. But how I would learn later that circumstance is a big part of life.

During those years, I couldn't count the tent revivals and church services that my dad led. We were always nearby with mom, either in the choir or congregation. One service took a new meaning for testimonies. It was called a "popcorn" service. Various people would stand from where they were seated and share a testimony. Everything seemed normal but then a little man stood to his feet and recited, "30 days hath September. April, June, and November." And he sat back down. Well, this caught everyone's attention. The service continued with others to share a quick testimony then the little guy stands again to recite, "Twinkle, twinkle little star. How I wonder what you are." A bit of silence fell. No one laughed but looked his way. It happened once more with his reciting, "Mary had a little lamb, who's fleece was white as snow." My dad with a smile on his face, regained everyone's attention with a congregational song. The little man just recited things he knew. Nothing more than random thoughts in his innocent mind. At least he had a support group that night.

Support groups of every kind are extremely important regardless of our background and especially when our minds begin to reflect change.

Now then, you can think what you want of nursing homes, but I believe them to represent another tower of strength.

They are strained with financial burdens that overshadow staffing, equipment, security, and all other activities that surround their needs. Staff assists in the overall care of the patient along with all unwanted chores. For me to think about the cleaning needs alone, it's massive.

My dad's sister-in-law was the Activities Coordinator at a nursing home for many years in our hometown. With her magnetic personality, she had a passion for serving her patients. She loved on those patients like no one else. She never cared about the constant interruptions; those little people came first to her. She always greeted them with a big hug and talked to them with compassion. She made them feel special. She made them feel like a person.

As I watched my mom become a shell of the person that she once was, we continued to treat her with utmost respect. That included speaking directly to her, saying hello to her, saying good morning and good night to her, bathing, changing her clothes, and feeding. We went through a phase where if I were in a conversation with someone while in her presence, she would babble loudly to be a part of the conversation. Many times, her babble would be so loud that I had to stop what I was saying; get down to her level, hold her hand and nod my head with her. She would respond with a big smile, nodding her head in return as if she understood she was a part of the conversation.

Navigation Check Point: Accounting and Valuables

- *<u>Banking</u>. They become very lax with paperwork, mail, and records. They may leave loose checks that are even signed laying around. It could be where they intended to pay a bill and then became distracted and just left the check. Be watchful of loose paperwork because those loose checks could fall into the wrong hands, even if in the trash. Properly destroy them and keep track of the numeric order of their checks.*

- *Accounts and Bills.* Yes, again, it's extremely important to watch their accounts for overdrawn banking, bills and statements. I helped my mom every Saturday and we would go through all of her mail together.
- *Power of Attorney.* While they may not be ready for someone to legally make decisions for them, a Power of Attorney should be in place for the unexpected that can occur at any time.
- *Lost and Found.* I discovered over time that mom had little hiding spots. I was careful to not draw attention to that fact but rather familiarized myself with those hidden areas (i.e., beneath a bed pillow, pant pockets, or between sofa cushions.) There were also times I found loose cash stuffed in the oddest places but have certainly found money stashed in magazines, cards, and Bibles. It's a good time to secure all valuables before they advance further along.

Early during her advancement, I began making notes and included the date for my own reference to track mom's progression. Understanding it's different in every case, I noticed there were definite changes with mom. I never really worried about it. One of the first things I did was to secure the bathroom and bedroom doors, so they did not lock. If they lock themselves in a room, it will be difficult explaining to them (behind a locked door) how to open the door. They become easily agitated and frustrated with any urgency and they do not handle excitement very well.

Baths will become a major hazard unless you have the proper safety measures in place. It is uncomfortable at first for both. Before extreme advancement, I would help mom into her bath and just stand outside the doorway to make sure she washed herself off and watched as she drained the water. She would use a towel to dry out as much in the bathtub before we stood her up. Over time, I placed a handrail on the tub, but note for caution, they can also be very dangerous. On a few occasions, mom had gripped the rail so tightly that she pulled it totally off.

While they can independently stay by themselves, they may call you frequently on the phone throughout the day and will most likely have the same conversation. They become very lonely. A lot of mom's calls would surround problems with the TV remote or discussion where she had mistakenly changed the channel or that the entire programming had become disarrayed. It is rather annoying to be interrupted so much over the simplest things, but you are their solid ground, and I would discourage missing a call from them in the event an accident has occurred.

Mom loved coffee but I noticed she would fall asleep so quickly even while holding a hot cup of coffee. Spills, stains, change of clothing begin to increase as does laundry. I kept mom independent as long as possible until trigger points introduced time for change. I believe they are relieved to know they have someone close to help them but as that happens, they become totally dependent on your assistance, and you must not walk away from them.

Coffee was a household item in our lives. You might have thought our lives even revolved around having coffee. Although mom loved coffee, it had a diuretic effect, and she would easily dehydrate. Since she didn't drink much of anything else, and with little activity, everything including her bowels were affected.

This is where our journey began to unfold (or unravel) regarding Alzheimer's. At that time, mom was sleeping in my room, but I had her in an oversized chair that was comfortable to her. I rather barricaded her into the chair, so it kept her safe from falling out of bed or getting up during the night without me hearing her.

<u>January 2017</u> It was around 3:00 a.m. when she was behaving erratic. I thought at first, she was dreaming but her movements and sounds were like none I had ever seen. I asked her if she was hurting. I couldn't get her to focus and respond.

> She was moaning and laughing at the same time with the behavior of one crying out for help but without control.

I called my brother Sammy first, to let him know I was calling for an ambulance. Once I notified emergency, I called my other brothers

Johnny and Steve. I slipped upstairs to let my sons, Justin and Jarod know and then waited for the ambulance. Once we arrived at the hospital, I called her sisters. I had no idea what to expect but knew that Sammy was on his way and that Johnny would be joining us later that day. We told Steve to wait in Nashville until we knew more.

After the nurse's initial reaction of "WOW" and her temperature reading of 104.7, it's no wonder that she was delirious! They fast approached the point of soaking her body to cool it down but soon whisked her away for scans. Initial reports were UTI and blocked bowel.

A deadly combination for sepsis.

Hours drug and we didn't even talk to one another apart from our lingered stares. We knew what the words were without speaking. That particular day was my birthday and I remember thinking, we would lose mom on my birthday and bury her on Sammy's. We only consoled one another during that 24-hour period. The ICU staff alerted us they would try a few manual attempts with procedures, but they were also very limited on what they could do and that her high fever complicated things even more. Her temperature did not want to lower and once sepsis developed, there would be a point of no return. I had never seen mom in such pain as to wail out for help, "SOMEBODY HELP ME!" We were soon motioned out.

Another 5 hours passed and a second manual attempt, then everything suddenly changed. We were called back in to see her and were shocked at the turnaround. We walked into her area and she immediately said, "well, there's my children!" with a big smile on her face. I used the same words the first nurse had said earlier, "WOW!"; as my brother and I stared at one another in amazement.

God had smiled on us.

> **Public Media Post**
> January 13, 2017
>
> Many, many thanks for the birthday greetings and wishes. It makes me feel very special! I love you guys!

What most don't know though, my family thought we were preparing to lose our most precious earthly treasure yesterday--mom.

But God in His great mercy and care always has a plan.

She remains in the hospital but has made a huge turnaround. I ask for continued prayers for her. Whereas I feared yesterday we might face saying goodbye soon, I am most thankful on this 56th birthday of mine that I got the best gift ever. Mom.

I must share a segment from my devotion today: Our Father is able to heal even the deadliest disease...when requesting restored health, we should ask with faith and trust.

James 5:14 Is any sick among you? let him call for the elders of the church; and let them pray over him,

Sometimes, we face a bad outcome. My family was bracing for the worst but allowing God to lead. I am grateful for my Christian family, and I fully understand we are all passing through this life journey. No one has the promise of tomorrow. Today may hold tragedy or triumph but I transfer it into the hand of Jesus who always brings peace. He offers real life beyond this world. Please remember a few of my close friends (unmentioned) as they ARE facing tragedies and goodbyes today and with a few others that are dealing with unknown outcomes.

To all of my family: the best I could ever give you are my prayers in return. When I read your posts and requests, I try to lift you up. Above all, keep the faith. Your prayer could be the difference in someone! We are really all just passing through!

The event certainly began an explosion that quickly led into Alzheimer's and the medical staff began to discuss the dementias with us. Alzheimer's doesn't always present in a sudden manner like we had seemingly experienced, but I believe combined with all other surrounding health issues, it seemed to be the major turning point with her in particularly. She was in the hospital for a couple of weeks and then transferred to a beautiful therapy facility for about a month and afterwards released home.

Then God smiled on us again.

My family. We didn't plan the flexibility with our schedules in staying with mom but at the time, Sammy had just retired, and Johnny was working through his retirement plans and recuperating himself from another major event. We could have never planned the timing, but the Lord orchestrated everything in His perfect time. I like to think that it's similar with the way the Lord planted that tree for Zacchaeus years before it was climbed.

The Lord knows our needs. Always.

Without batting an eye or even discussing a schedule, we began to rotate our days so mom would not be alone. We cared for her in different ways, but she had always loved us independently too. After she transitioned home, a physical therapist visited twice each week. Simple things like standing up from a chair became difficult. She was doing her best but would become easily frustrated if she could not do things quickly.

Mom initially showed some improvement but began a decline almost immediately at the end of therapy. Moving forward, we continued with routine doctor visits and my brothers arranged to stay with her during the day while I worked. We each worked with her to improve independence with standing, walking, and balance as the therapist had recommended but she was never able to regain full body control.

Personality changes became increasingly noticeable. We had many questions about behaviors with little insight. Still, we kept her moving as much as possible. Keeping her mobile and active, we continued with weekend visits with her sisters.

Navigation Check Point: Hygiene

- *Wardrobe*. Even though button down shirts seem like a great idea, I ended up using mostly sweatshirt pullovers for mom. They were soft, warm and easy to put on her. Button down garments I found to be a struggle because getting her arms in the sleeves had awkward pulls and tugs.
- *Bathing*. This is tricky and dangerous. You will find what works best but for us and as long as possible, I sat mom on the toilet (that had handles) and started with her hair. Then I disrobed her top, washed her off. Dried her upper body and placed clean clothes on her and then did her lower torso and legs in the same manner. It was tiring but it worked until she became bedridden and then thankfully, Hospice provided bathing assistance. There were many times obviously that I needed to bath her without the help of medical assistance. I just took my time and moved her very slowly.
- *Dental*. They may find it confusing to spit out toothpaste after a point. This was the case with mom. She would spit in the floor and then swallow mouthwash. I just did the best I could for her oral care.
- *Shoes*. I used a slide-on style with rubber soul for mom's shoes and also rubber-soul socks but discovered they were hard to find because they were seasonal. I did order online several types but it was difficult to gage sizing and proper style, and when they didn't properly fit, would be a waste of additional products.
- *Jewelry*. There's just no point. With the exception of a jeweled pin (which she loved) during the holidays, I would occasionally place something on her garment because I knew it was something mom would like, but otherwise, I reframed from placing jewelry on her.

Early on, there was no need for durable medical but gradually, we became in need of a walker. Mom was very awkward in getting up from a sitting position to the point of her pulling *us* down. She was incredibly strong. With her amazing strength, we grew stronger ourselves just to support her. She began to shuffle her feet when walking and that made her feet become easily entangled. I kept her in a soft slide shoe with rubber sole, but she would sometimes trip between the rubber sole and her shuffling feet. Her vision was fading more and more. She became afraid of minor things she saw, items hanging on the walls or distortions from the television screen.

While tracking this storm, we evaluated the items we might need on hand. I was fortunate to find two wheelchairs at a thrift store. One was a portable size and the other was fully equipped for everything, including a reclined position feature and a holder for an oxygen tank. Both were in excellent condition and looked brand new after cleaning them up. We also purchased a walker with a seat and assisted handlebars for the bathroom. We already had a standard walker and a portable toilet frame. We didn't need them right away but knew the day would quickly arrive.

Public Media Post
September 23, 2018

Those who answer the call with being caregivers for their parents or other loved ones can only understand my words here. You must learn to accept who they become.

They don't understand even the simple things like they've done though their lifetime. Like little ones, their skills are learning in ways they never have before. Only, their skills are fading.

They are learning to communicate and walk differently. They don't recognize as they once could. They will not be able to "grow" through these phases. If we could look toward their new tomorrow (in Christ), with where they are quickly moving...try to remain in that prospective because as Believers, that's where our eyes are to remain always. On the sky. On Christ alone.

It is extremely difficult (mentality and physically) and I know I cannot get through one single day without the Lord's help. I miss who my mom was and I miss the friendship we closely shared but I love her even more with who she is now. Innocent and purely in the moment. Her thoughts are rambling and her mind lives in the seconds. But we

> are still besties and the way she looks at me now is what I would describe as genuine trust. What an honor.
>
> Thank you for continuing prayers for my mother, Steve, Johnny, Sammy, Justin and Jarod (and all others I've not mentioned in my family) who are living this journey hand in hand as we keep our eyes on The One we genuinely trust day by day.
>
> Christ alone.

With dementias, each phase is a learning experience for everyone involved; both for the patient and the person assisting them. You would not think walkers could be dangerous, but they are. They will grab the walker as they begin to sit or stand expecting it to be stationary and as a result, they may have a hard fall while holding onto the walker. These little patients can have extremely tight grips too. Don't underestimate their strength even if they only weigh 100 lbs. or less.

I admit, many times, I found myself to be irritated with mom over the smallest things or simplest of tasks. I would blurt out, "come on mom…you can do that." I would quickly stop in my tracks when she would reply, "I'm sorry." I would apologize to her and get so frustrated at myself for being so inconsiderate to her. I apologized A LOT.

> But that's just part of the reality adjustments that unfolded before us.

I would raise my voice because her hearing increasingly began to fail. I had to raise my voice even louder to just keep her attention with what we were doing. If we walked down the hall, she would chatter all the way and be so distracted to the point we would both almost fall. I would shake her hands to get her attention and say, "MOM!

Pay attention! Let's walk!" She began to have a prominent lean in her body and I mean a *very strong lean forward*.

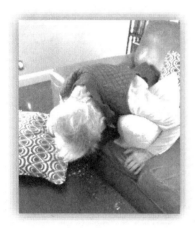

She wasn't dizzy, her body just leaned forward and she would press forward *with force*. It never made sense because she would go through patterns of time with it. One day would be extreme, the next day back to normal. There were days where she would lean so strongly even in a sitting position and she would have her head completely resting in her lap. We could never explain that behavior. We did our best to secure her further but there was absolutely no control in keeping her upright on those days, walking or sitting. We had heard that people can have multiple dementias at once and we wondered if this were effects of Parkinson's or Lewy Bodies. I learned myself to walk backwards while holding both of her hands in order to watch her body position and balance. Between her chatter, attention span, distractions and body position, we had to learn to adjust our own body reactions so we could catch her at any given time. Keeping her on her toes; kept US on OUR toes.

She began another little habit that honestly, I believe if she were hanging off a cliff, her fingers would sustain her on the edge. The pinch of her fingers would grab things so tightly that we would need to pry, whatever it was, out of her hands. This could be clothing or grabbing someone's hand as they walked by. The friends that would stop by to visit my sons would always stop to speak with her. She would undoubtedly hold onto them in some fashion and I would need to step in and pry her fingers lose. She had become a bit of a flirt and we laughed about her wanting to hang on to those boys. The guys had such a sweet nature around her too and her eyes would sparkle around them. She kept a crush on Sammy though.

She also began to chatter non-stop in a rocking motion. It didn't matter if we were part of the chatter conversation or not. It was rhythmic too and would sound like a chant. She would many times become out of breath because she would repeat it quickly and over and over; sometimes for hours at a time and even throughout an entire day.

> Her hands trembled and in holding them, you could feel the presence of a tremor. I imagined that was exactly what was going on inside her mind in an uncontrollable manner.

Her attention span was essentially in the seconds, and I watched her mind transition into split-seconds. There was no more following along in our conversation. We would call out to her and she would answer in one-word sentences.

Our family planned to meet at our family church that year for her birthday and Mother's Day. She was not able to enjoy being there but had instead became so troubled that it was disruptive to everyone in the congregation. It was non-stop chatter, crying and calling out my name, "Donna!" She would call out to Sammy in a loud manner while he was leading the sermon. You could see the fear in her eyes. I think she knew where she was, but she could not be quiet or still. Even after the service, our family had lunch together at the church and she cried the entire time. The moment we left in the car; she immediately settled. She was terrified that day because of the large open space and being surrounded by people. People that she knew and loved just a short time earlier but presently within her mind, it was just too overwhelming. The car ride calmed her, because it was a small, confined area. It reminded me of an infant when they are unsettled, and we can relax them with pacifiers or bottles. We're not able to do that with our aging folks. They are simply not able to communicate as they once could. They are frustrated. They are afraid. Everything around them seems loud and unfamiliar. But, like swaddling a baby into a blanket, she immediately settled back into her little world once we secured her into the car.

Psalm 61:2

When my heart is overwhelmed; lead me to the Rock that is higher than I.

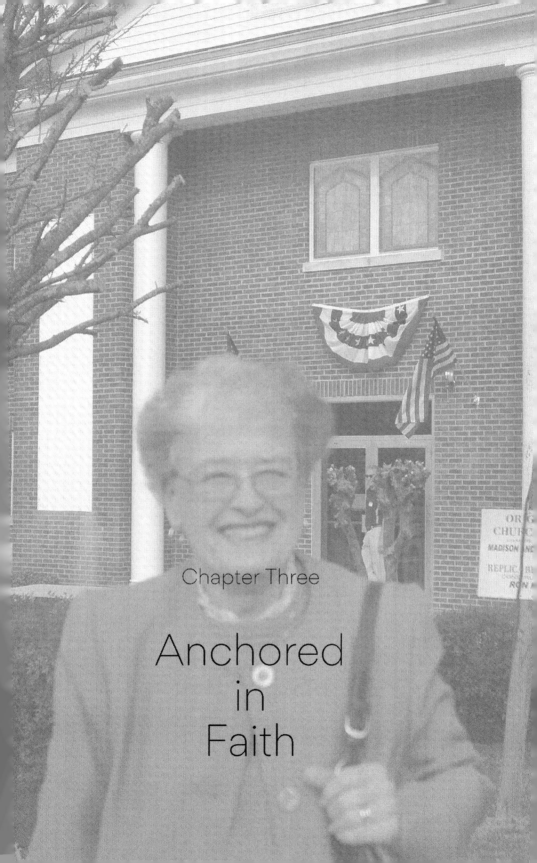

Chapter Three

Anchored in Faith

The emotions and impact from the effects of Alzheimer's are deeper than the ocean. Like the tide, it rolls in regardless, sinking your feet immediately into the sand while at the same time pulling you out to sea. The undertow is strong, and…

> …you will exhaust yourself trying to fight for your loved one as who they once were.

The water submerges them away from their past. You find yourself getting to know a new personality that bobs back and forth like a deep-sea buoy. Endurance will become your permanent dock and you will need unwavering faith to sustain these winds.

Where on this earth do you get THAT?

While in elementary school, my sixth-grade science teacher assigned everyone a project and wanted us to find pictures that were descriptive of a different assigned word to everyone. My assigned word was "Endurance." I had to ask mom what she thought about that word and she suggested that I find a picture from a magazine of someone working physical labor. I've thought a lot about that word over the years.

Endurance.

Surely, it must have been assigned to me as it would apply to my life in the years ahead.

While witnessing the destructive disease that mom's sister Lee had endured with Alzheimer's, mom had prayed many times and worried that she herself would come face-to-face with the ugly disease. Just a few years earlier, she had repeatedly prayed and asked the Lord to prevent her from getting the disease because she saw the devastation that it took on her sweet sister. We would visit her in the facility on occasions and leave in tears after every visit. It got so emotionally hard for mom to see her in that condition that (right or wrong) I stopped taking her there but rather kept in contact with her other sister Clellene about her care. As mom continued to worry about herself becoming struck with the disease, I could only assure her that we would take care of her regardless.

Now, wait just one minute here.

Why would the Lord NOT answer her specific prayer about this?

She had lived a faithful Christian life so why would God permit something so ugly to become so prominent the last few years of her life? It's the same answer I have for children that suffer from child abuse or neglect.

> I have no idea. I will just never understand it.

I've entered many conversations about it. Why *does* the Lord allow bad things to happen to good people? People have written books about it. People have researched it. People have complained to God about it. To Believers in Christ, one of history's most recognized conversations took place between Job and God. Job didn't have Alzheimer's (or at least the Bible doesn't reference it) however, Job *was* stricken with boils from head to toe. Talk about physical pain. His own wife told him to curse God and die. That's putting things in perspective after the Lord allowed his entire family and farmlands to be totally destroyed.

The culprit behind the scenes? Satan himself.

True, Job was a man of God, yet the Lord allowed these things to happen to him. The book of Job describes Satan asking God for permission to test and destroy Job. As the story unfolds through the catastrophes, it's just like us to naturally dwell on what he lost but let's focus for a minute on his faith.

He was anchored in faith.

The Lord allowed essentially anything to happen apart from his life to be taken. I challenge you to look it up in the Bible and read it all for yourself (*Job 1:1-19; 2:7; 9 and 42:12*). The Lord protected his life and fully restored him and blessed him even more than before because of his faithfulness during the events that played out.

How does this relate to Alzheimer's? Job's series of unfortunate events has nothing to do with my current situation, right? Let's be honest, don't you feel better when you hear that someone else is going through situations much worse than you?

Is your world crashing down?

Bankruptcy?

Divorce?

Unexpected job loss?

Health concerns?

And what do we do at that point? Give up?

Unfortunately, many do. Yet God in His great mercy, cares deeply for us and provides us with unfailing hope amid our catastrophes.

I believe that to be the worst tragedy of all; not to accept how the Lord cares for us. We are to blame for isolating ourselves apart from Him. Living through these horrific life events is overwhelming. Trust me, I know. I've had my share. You will experience great trials on this earth and how you "get back up" is everything. There is no greater confidence and peace that you will experience during those times as when the Lord is with you.

The Lord was with Job.

Speaking about myself now, there was a time in my life that I realized if He were present in Job's life, He would be present in my life too. I just needed to ask. If God's Word was REALLY true, then He could deliver me from whatever attack I was under. I believed that the Bible was true. I believed that the Lord existed. And the Lord began to conclude in my heart that He could deliver me too.

My prayer? That literal miracle prayer: "help me Lord!"

Bankruptcy. Bankruptcy was one of the most degrading realities in my life while simultaneously combatting a divorce. The Lord carried me through the tangled debris field and with determination and hard work, He enabled me to effectively refinance my home and successfully "grow" through the circumstance without it destroying my life. It was a devastating failure, but God led me through the fires without being singed.

Divorce. I swore I would never remarry after my first marriage of two years at a young age. But of course, I did and gratefully, my second marriage produced two of the most wonderful children I could ever ask for. The Lord certainly knew I needed my boys. I am blessed with each and would not trade them for the world. I am so proud of them.

Unfortunately, after 15 years of marriage, this divorce delivered scars for us all. Thankfully, through prayer and God's grace, He carried us through a most unexpected and traumatic journey that continued 15 years AFTER the divorce. This being my greatest challenge, I was at dead end and had to truly learn to place it all in the Lord's hands. Colossians 1:17 became my cornerstone. *And He is before all things and by Him all things consist.* Everything else in my life had crashed. I was at rock bottom.

Rock bottom is not over in a couple of weeks. It is a despairing season. I'm speaking in terms of my heavy burdens, not casting down or placing blame on others. It has been a torrential storm. My heart has not been fully capable of expressing anything into words, **but God**, holds us each in His nail-scarred hands. Psalm 147:3 says, "He heals the brokenhearted and binds up their wounds." That's us. ALL of US. Personally, it taught me true dependence on God and on that note, I give all glory to Him.

Unexpected job change. After moving through the bankruptcy, divorce and doing the best I could with single parenting, my job was suddenly placed as temporary status amid refinancing my home from the previous battles. Incredibly and out of nowhere, a new job opened up in the best possible direction and in the *same day* that I was offered that job, I received information that my application loan had been approved and I needed to sign the papers on *the same day*. Only the Lord can orchestrate those events because I had literally no control over each scenario.

Health concerns. Growing older introduces many health concerns. Rheumatoid arthritis, arthritis, osteoarthritis, bursitis….whatever "itis" existed, I felt like it was attacking my body. In fact, I found myself most days feeling like I'd been trampled by a team of horses before I got out of bed in the morning. You know, morning stiffness, aches and pains. Mom and I would frequently joke in years past about going to bed with BEN and waking up with ARTHUR *(Bengay and arthritis)*. And of course, there is diabetes and heart disease. The thing is, enduring health trials, and many more health concerns not even mentioned here, the Lord brought me through each one. Most times, I would be pressed against all odds where He would be the ONLY one that could deliver me. While enduring these battles, He began to reveal to me that when I leaned on Him, I was getting to know Him more personally and witness more of His unlimited power. He is Omnipresent and Omnipotent. What is documented in

God's Word through those "Bible stories" as we like to say…is truth and can be applied to our lives today. I ask you two simple questions:

Do you believe in God?

Do you believe that the Bible is Truth?

If your answer is no, I encourage you then to reach out to Him deep within your heart. No one else even needs to know at this point. It's all personal between you and Him. He holds us all accountable for our own decision though. So, don't let it cost your eternity!

If your answers are yes, why then, would the Lord present Truth for us to only perceive it as a "good story?"

No, it doesn't stop there.

When I look back over my life, I have truly had a great life. And like everyone else, I have also made a lot of mistakes with many lessons learned. It's been through those mistakes that I would turn to my Bible devotions for encouragement.

> Was I turning to Him or was He calling me to Him? Does He use our failures to reach us?

Absolutely.

And God gives you the freedom to decide for yourself. He won't force you to do anything. But He does call you. He yearns for you. He promises to guide you through any situation in life. We must be willing to trust Him though. If I shared with you my deepest struggles, you would say I'd been charred through circumstance. However, I'm not a product of my circumstances. I am a product of my own decisions, good or bad. I accept that and I'm really no different than anyone else. In some cases, I brought on situations by making bad decisions. In other cases, I've purely been under attack.

Likened to Job though, God brought beauty from my charred ashes.

The good news for me is that He's not done with me yet. I only need to place my trust in Him daily. I do trust that the Lord has higher reasons that we may not understand until we reach our heavenly home. But it really won't even matter then. There's really only ONE decision that matters in this life and that is this: Do you trust Christ as Lord in your life or not?

Navigation Check Point: Eternity

So, it all comes down to this, with me writing this book. It's not about me at all. And it's really not even about mom. But, it's all about YOU and your eternity. Please, if you glean nothing else from my writings but this, I urge you to listen with your heart to what God is saying to you now.

- *<u>Sin</u>. At the fall of man and when sin entered this world (Genesis 3:6), the earth became cursed and all therein (Genesis 3:7-19). Because God is perfect and cannot look upon sin, God took the first blood sacrifice to cover the sin for the atonement with Adam and Eve (Genesis 3:21).*
- *<u>Savior</u>. Since sin had entered the world, there was separation from God and the wages of sin is death (Romans 6:23). The Lord knew we needed a Savior. We are therefore born into this sinful world (Romans 3:23) and are not able to save ourselves (Ephesians 2:9). God is Holy and must punish sin but provided for us a Savior (John 14:6). Jesus, God's Son, provides us forgiveness of our sins as He died on the cross for all sin (1 Peter 3:18); then was resurrected for our justification (Romans 4:25). This is our only Hope (John 1:12) but the choice is ours. He doesn't force us. It is of your own free will. He does call us to decide though. No response is a response and your eternal mistake.*
- *<u>Confess</u>. Although salvation is a gift from God (Ephesians 2:8), we must understand that we are of sin and must confess our sin (Acts 3:19). This doesn't mean just feeling sorry for our sin, yet instead turning to God through Jesus and turning away from our sin (Acts 26:20). The Bible says "Whosoever calls upon the name of the Lord shall be saved (Romans 10:13)." You only need to ask the Lord to save you. Based on God's Word, you can follow this simple prayer:* **God, I know that I am a sinner and cannot save myself. I believe that Jesus died on the cross for my sin and was raised from the dead. I know I need forgiveness for my sin and need Your forgiveness through Christ. I want to trust and follow You as my Savior.**
- *<u>Accept</u>. Standing on the Word of God in confessing your sin, you have accepted God's gift of eternal life through Jesus. God keeps His promise! You have repented of your sin (Acts 3:19); have placed your faith in Jesus Christ (Ephesians 2:8-9) and God has heard your prayer! Remember! Whoever calls upon the Lord shall be saved. He has recorded your name eternally in heaven (Luke 10:20) and your salvation can never be taken away (Hebrews 6:4-6). Share your new salvation with others! I encourage you to read His Word, find a church and let Him work through you in amazing ways.*

Jesus was the only One who brought genuine peace in my life and I am eternally grateful that mom personally introduced me to Him. One of the highest compliments she ever gave to me was one evening after sharing a devotion together, she looked up to me and said, "you teach me so much." WOW. I was astounded by that comment. She is the one that I have admired my entire life, the one who taught me everything and yet paid me such a compliment. Jesus was what mom's life was about. What a difference Christ can make out of anyone's chaos. And once you experience His unwavering hand amid life storms, you will understand more and more why Job kept anchored in his faith.

> ## Public Media Post
> March 1, 2019
>
> Rain. It can be symbolic.
>
> Some days and very unpredictably, I get to my office, close the door and cry for a minute. Even though it can linger on and off all day, for the most part, it is but a brief release of emotion.
>
> It is a definite release though that my body actually needs. I really don't even like to cry...it makes my eyes swell and let's face it, as we age...it's all the worse. For the most part I'm a closet crier but for now there is this ever constant reminder that one day, mom will be gone. I think this overbearing emotion comes from several areas.
>
> Not being able to have a complete conversation with my best friend. Asking for her advice. Sharing a funny moment together. Cooking together. Premature grief. Pure exhaust both mentally and physically. Thank the Lord for my family, friends and coworkers who understand and let me cry on their shoulders too. Just like all other seasons in life, this too shall pass and I have found that most want to share their own stories but offer it with

encouragement. The impending and looming reality is very hard to walk masked with a smile and strength ALL of the time.

The truth is, without prayers from my family and friends, I would have washed away with all this dreary rain long ago. We just can't face a thing without the Lord holding us together. So, if you should see me wailing up with tears in my eyes, I'm ok.

I'm ok because my Father has me. It's ok to cry too....I just don't dwell there and I don't advise anyone to dwell there. Somewhere....and yes....maybe even over the rainbow....He has a greater purpose. And that's exactly what I want to be a part of.

Oh yeah, and to my family, friends and coworkers....I always covet your prayers and great big hugs!

Romans 8:28

And we know that all things work together for good to them that love God, to them who are the called according to His purpose.

Chapter Four

Dynamics

Through my personal experiences, my advice is that you best be anchored in SOMETHING because as a caregiver, the reality swells like a tidal wave. You see something ahead but it's deceivingly at a safe distance. You believe you have good footing on the shore, but the sand gives away quickly with the tide and suddenly, you're swept away with a whole new set of emotions and responsibilities that you've never experienced before. With this progression, your life, dwelling, and existence becomes unrecognizable to what it once was.

Entering through the doors of a caregiver's home is not pretty. If mom had the words now that once described my belongings and personal space, it would have been everything had its place. I once loved color schemes, holiday decorating, rearranging rooms with furniture, lighting, and personal treasures. That desire flew out my window sometime back due to the new and unexpected responsibilities. That was a part of me that I enjoyed, and I certainly didn't expect an attitude of "I don't care" anymore. Between work and activity that surrounds life obligations, there is naturally a degree of disorder. Even so (and still), I like order but was reminded then how I was forced to let the tidy things go from my life. It was like I was living with young children again with bins of toys scattered about that you try to disguise in baskets. How though, with adult items, do you find essential area and space for the adult diapers, wipes, and etc.? We were offered a sling style lift harness for mom when she became bed-ridden that we tried out for a while but honestly, I chose to return it shortly after because it was just another huge piece of equipment, and it took about 30 minutes of my extra time to properly secure the harness into place around her. For some, it might be the very life-saver device that works for your family. It just didn't work for me. I was still exhausted after transporting her from bed to toilet and visa-versa.

Things certainly become complex with adulthood. I remember simpler days in my youth, when we had one bathroom closet that we tossed all of our dirty clothes in. We didn't even have a laundry basket; the floor of the closet was just always filled with dirty clothes, sometimes to the point that we couldn't close the closet door. Dirty towels would be heaving beyond its space. Our laundry room at that time was an outdoor utility room which is almost unheard of these days. Today, people create beautiful laundry room "areas" that I can only wish were a part of my world. Why the sudden talk about laundry?

Because the reality is for both a caregiver's world *and* for laundry, it is very time consuming, smelly, dirty and no one likes doing it. You must sort it, wash it, dry it and then put it away. At any given time, I have a dirty hamper filled with dirty clothes (and most likely damp with mildew), with clothes found in both the washer and dryer. Our clothes rarely even make it to the closet and drawer stage. As adults, we learn to wear and (hopefully) wear it again before it needs cleaned. But in taking care of another adult that has uncontrollable functions, there will be days that a change of clothes is required twice and even three times per day due to accidents. Spills are one thing, but accidents are another. You must remember they are not able to control body functions nor are they capable of even saying anything at a certain stage. Believe me, it's hard. Loving through this ugly beast of Alzheimer's.

| Love is a choice though. |

Like the changes that surround your family, massive dynamics are also changing inside your loved one. You care for this person unmeasurably and of course there is love. However, watching your loved one go through such a difficult and uncontrollable transition is heart wrenching. I totally understand that all families and situations are different, and most are not able to care for a loved one 24/7 because of other responsibilities. I get that. Our independent adult lives are packed full of daily necessities apart from the added burdens of caregiving. Your loved one might sense the added burden on you and relieve you from checking in on them with comments like, "it's ok, I know you're working and very busy…"

Their days are long though. Every day is long, and then it's day after day of the same thing in their world. They forget when the mail is delivered. They forget how to operate simple things such as a microwave. I know mom had difficulty seeing the buttons on our microwave and I placed (don't laugh, it worked) an adhesive foot corn pad (it was all I had at the time) onto the 30 second button so she could feel the placement and not set the microwave for something crazy like a setting of 30 minutes! Our days have certainly been tested and it was hard to keep love in mind when things became so challenging; both physically and mentally for each of us. Many times, I found my own behavior acting out like an ugly beast. I am a highly patient person by nature but my patience had been tested and tried; run over, backed-over, soaked, wrung out and drained through a tube-wringer.

Before our caregiving roles became 24/7 and while she was able to stay alone during the day by herself, being attentive to her immediately when I walked in from work was very important. We would all come and go through the day which brought activity around her but having one-on-one communication was major. Besides, recognize that we all need one another and crave love and appreciation at all levels.

Navigation Check Point: Environment

During early transition, please consider these things:

- *Rugs. Mom shuffled her feet when walking so I removed all area rugs to decrease exposure to falls.*
- *Door locks. I removed the locked doorknobs from my bedrooms and bathrooms. You can consider securing the top of entrance doorways in case they become a "runner" and wander off which is a very real issue.*
- *Lighting. My home did not have a great deal of natural light and mom had poor vision. I used mirrors to reflect more light in areas that I could. I also changed bulbs to bright white.*
- *Heat and Air. Their body temperatures are naturally colder because they are certainly not active. I had a few toss blankets but discovered mom would let them fall onto the floor and that became a fall hazard. Instead, I layered her clothing with sweaters. I also draped one around her neck like a shawl and let her hands hold onto the sleeves.*
- *Land Lines. While she was still independent, I used a land line with pictures on speed dial that was programed according to the person in the photo. They make multiple calls and will likely to discuss the same conversation as before.*
- *Television. They will have difficulty using a remote. I kept a picture of my remote with me to help her identify the buttons when she called me with questions.*

- *Microwave. I used adhesive raised stickers to place over the 30 second start button because mom could not see the front panel to read the difference, nor could she determine the time difference in use.*

I found myself many times though fighting through a multitude of many other emotions.

There's just no escaping it.

> You don't have the freedom to do anything apart from tending to your caregiver duties.

When I struggled just to move her from her bed onto the portable toilet and then to her wheelchair, I would be exhausted. She was too. She resisted every movement. I'm not sure if it was painful for her. We wondered that many times. If so, she never indicated it in any manner. But she relaxed once settled into her personal space again.

My brothers and I handled her in different ways, as you would in caring for a baby. I would position myself with my legs straddling the wheels of her wheelchair (which was quite a stretch); unstrap her safety belt, embrace her with my arms extended beneath her armpits (as if I were going to front-on bear-hug her) and lift her to stand up slowly. I did my best to be cautious of lifting because of my lower back and sciatica issues. Once I had her in a standing position, I could hold onto her and help her begin to slowly walk while holding her hands tightly, still rather locked arm in arm. When the stage came where she could no longer walk, I would stand her up to transfer her onto the toilet, hug her tightly (again, with our bodies front to front embraced) and then reach with one arm around to pull down her clothing to sit her onto the toilet. Many times, just while sitting her onto the toilet, everything would miss, meaning another entire clean up.

When there were incidents of bowel movements or urine leaks onto clothing, we obviously needed to clean her up and change her clothing. There are flushable adult wipes available, and you will likely go through one entire pack for these incidents. I certainly kept those on hand but ended up just using the baby wipes because of expense with the amount that is needed. Again, we are talking adult strength and size of these incidents. Many times, I would need to even mop the floors because of the waste amount and scurry that surrounded the mess. Because of the heap, I just tossed everything into a garbage bag for disposal rather than flush because of the volume. You don't want to deal with sewage backups along with what you are already facing.

Apart from any sewage talk, there are always foul aromas. Enough said and I think you know why. I hope that paints enough of a visual picture of moving her around for restroom necessities.

Walking can really be dangerous. My home was rather small and that was likely good because distance was short. There were no stairs we had to contend with inside my home while walking with her but once she was constrained to a wheelchair, we had to use ramps over my front door entrance and that was so very difficult. I was grateful for the ramps because we could not do without them. I think my muscles grew strong enough that I felt I could lift the side of a car! Her wheelchair alone seemed to weigh 100+ pounds and my entranceway was on a hillside and at an angle, so it was very tricky and added around 30 minutes extra time in just loading everything into the vehicle. Let me tell you, I was exhausted by the time I got into the car.

We all had an opinion about what she may or may not have felt from pain in moving her around either. We were close enough to discuss it openly but many times we resisted our own feelings about it because it hurt us to think we might be inflicting more physical pain to her. On an average day, when she could walk with assistance, we tried to walk her to the restroom four times during the day and evening. By that stage, I kept her in heavy strength overnight pull-ups. There is a period before they need assistance in walking that they need to go to the restroom once or twice during the night. This means, you should be ready at any hour to assist. Average sleep patterns for the caregiver are like having a newborn baby; you are awakened about every hour. At least that's what I experienced.

> It was very easy to let the emotion control our own thoughts and actions.

Much over my life, I made decisions based on my emotions at the time. I never recommend that. I recognize now that the Lord has used this journey to mold me. Regardless, I've had to be submissive to His lead and I believe that is where genuine maturity begins; being submissive and obedient to His will.

When you open your home to others, all dynamics change. Including routines, children, behaviors, pets and all other aspects of typical living arrangements. Don't get me wrong, I love my family. We are close. But it brings about change and it's important to remember it's just as difficult on the others that come and go from your home. You must decide sleeping arrangements, meals, laundry (including bedding), room temperatures, etc. What are they trading for this too? In other words, it makes an impact in their normal routine and other extended families. There are new schedules to work around, temperaments, and likes and dislikes of what may have been a normal routine. Not to sound childish but our center discussions were similar to the daily report you would receive from a day care facility with a toddler.

What was her mood?

What did she eat?

Did she have a bowel movement?

Privacy flies out the window.

You learn to keep track of bathroom trips and honestly, plan around them. Can you imagine, as an adult, waiting for someone to help you get to the bathroom? And yet, they are literally at someone's mercy to help assist. I managed to line the inside of her portable potty with a garbage bag and then used spare diaper pull-ups inside to catch the debris. It was easier to clean up and keep the aroma subtle. In between your daily duties, planning around these trips come around the clock. The goal is to also have them relieve themselves while on the toilet. Most times, that does not occur. Think of a toddler in potty training. You go often to have them learn the routine but to the aging folks with dementia, they don't retain the behavior. They become more and more dependent on you and of course, they eventually lose all control. Most bathroom breaks took at least 20 minutes to (believe it or not) an hour. You walk slowly with them and if they are in a wheelchair, you still have the transport and the adjustments of their clothing in moving them back and forth.

I tried to keep mom on an average mealtime routine, but their appetite is different too. I wondered if mom's body just went through the motions and habits of eating. Because of the small portions they begin to ingest, we would offer soft cereal bars and ice cream sandwiches in between a meal. It was hard to find a happy medium because of the frequent behavior modifications. I learned her little habit of putting her finger in her mouth if she was hungry or she would bite on the stuffed animal's ear that we kept in her hands. Their hands draw and become so tightly closed; you need to have them grasp something soft to prevent their fingers from locking. Mealtimes take anywhere between 30 minutes to an hour. Eating for them is very slow and you have to constantly coax them to take another bite, chew, and 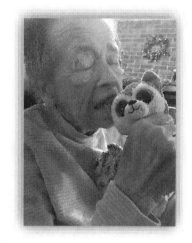 swallow; just like a toddler. They take small bites and chew a long time to the point that the food (if served warm) would no longer taste good to you or me. I've even wondered about their taste buds. I've seen mom's taste behaviors change. Certainly, be aware of instant choking or coughing on their food. Mom would hold food in her mouth without our even knowing at times. That is very dangerous especially at bedtime.

It was nice for me to be around my brothers again under one roof. And it was good for my children to have that extended environment of family within our home. We all had to adjust our lives on this path. During a particular period, my oldest was an officer and worked third shift. We had to learn to adjust our sounds during the day while he slept and likewise, we would hear him during the night while he cooked pizza on his nights off. The 3:00 a.m. aroma filled the house, and the smell would wake me from my dead sleep. My youngest would come and go between school, work and his campus life. My front yard resembled a small car lot at times, and we constantly needed to adjust our car line up to the order of the day. I found myself needing to stop by the grocery store a lot more. There was a difference in the use of products, increased use of them, and the added budget and fluctuating cost. We had trouble during 2020 because of the widespread panic with supply and demand on paper products and cleaners. Who would have guessed we would experience that at all? I special ordered heavy duty overnight adult diapers and the boxes were huge. We received boxes of diapers and bed pads from Hospice that were all needed but I had to find the extra space for the large, bulky boxes.

Many times, I felt guilty in leaving my brothers during the day. While mom's mind was racing with periods of her crying, I knew the days were long for my brothers. As she grew farther and farther away in her mind and habits, the day was easier to accept. I still felt bad though in leaving. Will she pass before I got home? Would it be tonight? Would we lose our own balance with her getting her into bed?

Our own minds traveled in many directions every single day. Oh, the dynamics of it all. Be prepared. Be very prepared.

> My heart slowly submerged in my own tears and drowned into a sea of despair between memory and emotion.

Yet once again, the water was insignificant to me for my love for her had drowned with the innocence of this soul.

And even though this journey was not what we would have chosen, Christ never left our side. Through it all, He grew my faith and I consistently learned to lean on Him more and more. That's exactly what He wants you know. That's the "mold" I mentioned earlier. He was molding me to lean on Him. His yoke is easy, and His burden is light (Matthew 11:28-30). You sure couldn't ask for a better Captain on your vessel. He knows the direction of the winds and the depth of your despair. I soon began to understand just how badly I needed Him and grew to depend on Him more and more. I thought my heart could not hold up to any more storms in life; and it couldn't…but what His hand sustained me. The prayers from my circle of family and friends were my lifeline. I truly felt their prayers.

I'm not sure why we treat prayer as a helpless and last resort either. Prayer is our greatest weapon. It was the prayers of others that held me up during this storm. Please remember that when someone asks for you to pray for them or if you offer upfront to pray for someone, take it literal. You are lifting them up to the Throne and it is in His control at that point forward.

Don't constrain God and His Omnipotent power even if you don't see immediate results in your prayers. We don't know His higher plan (which is always best).

By the way, our prayers don't have expiration dates.

And, if you feel you have no one to lean on in praying for you, rest in this: Christ Himself, prayed for YOU in the garden (John 17:20-21).

So, do you see? Our prayers never expire!

2 Corinthians 12:9

And He said unto me, My grace is sufficient for thee; for My strength is made perfect in weakness.

Chapter Five

Submerged in Who They Become

We certainly found ourselves getting acquainted with a new mom and yet I found myself falling deeper in love with this new person because of her pure innocence. We constantly found ourselves looking for logic in her behaviors, but in my opinion, logic does not apply to anyone's behaviors with Alzheimer's. However, it excels as a guessing game each new day. You eventually accept that the person you once knew, has drifted away.

> There is a new person that you've been introduced to yet without formal introductions. One day, you just find yourself submerged in who they've become. Oh, how I dreaded this voyage.

Personally, my heartache in losing mom began at that introduction phase with her and swept me through the stages of grief before she even passed. When she did pass (October 24, 2020), I confess that I experienced great relief. It's hard for me to even admit my relief because I felt somewhat guilty and even still that I did not do enough or that I should have done things differently.

I observed that while someone enters the different stages and levels of dementia, they may recognize that their behavior isn't right. They sense something is wrong beyond their control, but they may also find ways to disguise it.

They can provoke conversations about different scenarios they've encountered. I'm not sure if it's a silent cry for help or if they are trying to determine if anyone notices anything different. Maybe both. The oddities may be as simple as stuffing tissues everywhere but excusing it away as padding that came with an item. This obviously makes no common sense whatsoever. But that is a small description of just ONE instance in a million.

Public Media Post
November 21, 2018

It's only natural to reflect during the holidays. This year, I sit surrounded by change. God's grace still allows us to have mom with us but as our family continues to expand and in different directions, we are, for the first time in my 57 years, not together during this Thanksgiving season as a family. For the most part over the years, we would celebrate on the actual holiday but as I tell my boys, whenever we are together...whatever day it us...is our holiday. I remember all of our holidays on Sharon Drive. It would be standing room only and we never knew who would show up. We always burned the rolls. This year, I will most likely forget they are even in the freezer. Oh sure, I have the double layer pumpkin pie, pecan pie, sweet potato casserole and my classic cranberry chutney (I think I'm the only one who loves) and even now as I'm waiting on the food to cook, I write this to clear my heart and mind. I also hear the babbling words from mom in the next room as she drifts off to sleep. Oh, the memories we share. I'm glad I did not realize that last year.... would; could have; in fact...be the last year my whole family might be together. My heart accepts this as God's grace. We would be too sad if last year we had known change would knock on our door so soon. We only need to trust God for all tomorrows.

In our family, whoever talks the loudest...has the floor. Needless to say: We. Are. Loud. Football playing on TV. Kids playing football outside. Kids playing football inside. Tight hugs and kisses. Mapping out our Black Friday plans. Drawing names within our family. The house being so stinking hot from continuous cooking for the previous 24 hours. Maybe 3 good hours of sleep because we squeeze every moment together laughing and talking. But this year....we begin a new path. It will be good. But I miss my family. I miss my brothers. I miss my sisters. I miss my nieces. I miss my nephews. I miss my great nieces and nephews. I miss the chaotic loud conversations. I even miss the hot house that between East TN weather and thermostats we could never properly regulate. But mostly, I miss my mom. I think it's good that while she is still here, change pays us a visit this Thanksgiving because things will never really be the same. God is easing us into the next chapter of life perhaps.

Yet, I praise Him in this change. He is so gracious. His love for me is unmeasurable. He has blessed my family. He has given me the best family in the world and it just keeps getting better because, we will eternally be together too. We are all a Christian family. We follow Christ. I am still surrounded by my loving extended family this Thanksgiving and I am grateful and thankful for them all. Wow. My heart is overwhelmed with true Thanksgiving. Even when change comes to visit. Open the door. Embrace the change. This journey has really just begun.

 I am forever grateful. Thanksgiving is exactly where you are...who you are with...and with gratefulness in your heart. Happy Thanksgiving to you all!

It was Christmas season just a few years earlier than these writings and mom carried around this small trinket that she had already given me years before. I was in the same room wrapping presents and she spotted the trinket on the dresser. She knew that we were preparing to exchange gifts and wanted to participate. She carried the little jewel around with her for a while and then abruptly asked me to hold out my hand. She simply said, "I want you to have this as a gift." She was so very sweet with her gesture and words,

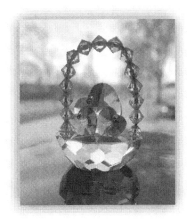

but it was her tenderness that pierced my heart. I'm not sure who needed that act of kindness the most. Me. Or, mom. The giver or the receiver. I will tell you that it sits in my window seal at my office now. No one else would give it second thought. But it is precious to me, and I remember the manner in which she presented it to me much more than when she originally gave it to me. It was moments as such that became golden. Be attentive with those tender moments because like the days with raising children, time passes quickly.

Music was the heart of her soul, and she would smile the biggest when we sang hymns and especially songs about Jesus' love. A simple yet utterly true song that, more than likely, we all learned in our childhood days. After singing, she would nod her head and say, "yes, yes" while smiling ear to ear.

I took her out as often as possible. Once we settled in the car, I would put a CD of her favorite music on to play while we drove, and she absolutely loved it. She would just sit there and smile so big that it reached across the car and made my heart smile. During the dementia days, those times brought laughter in our hearts for sure.

All of their emotions are extremely heightened. Highs and lows of both extremes; they literally live in the moment, so time is of no essence to them.

> Their affection is basic and simple, and it makes you understand even more that the simple things are what mean the most in life.

Mom kept her physical abilities until her major turning point in January 2017 although even before, there were typical aging behaviors with changes in her concentration.

While elderly but still somewhat independent, she would dress herself in pajamas at bedtime, and then most mornings, she would already be fully dressed before my feet hit the floor. I'm not sure what time during the night she would slip back into her clothes; I would subconsciously listen for her even while I slept. Often, her clothes would be backwards, and I figured out over time that her focus would be on the garment tag. When getting dressed, she knew the tag belonged in the back, so her attention was totally on the tag. I did my best to make light of any situation because you never really want to alarm or embarrass them.

Navigation Check Point: Activities

Like a toddler, their hands are constantly roaming but not in a learning manner. A toddler will grow through their experiments, a senior is simply restless.

- *Flute and Harmonica.* I kept a harmonica and wooden flute handy for mom. She would see them on the table in front of her and actively use them. It exercised her mind and provided a little exercise for her lungs. It certainly provided entertainment for everyone around her. Johnny also taught her to whistle again.
- *Toys and Photos.* Small toys for babies can also stimulate senior skills. Bright colors, zippers and pulls help calm their fidgety hands. I also kept a wallet style photo album that she could easily carry and filled it with family photos.
- *Busy Blankets.* Busy blankets are on the market for Dementia patients, but they are easily made from a pillow sham and fastening/stitching simple items to the sham. It provides visual stimulation and keeps their hands active.
- *Jingle Bells.* A great activity during the day and I also used for mom's clothing at night in order to hear her if she tried to get up without me knowing.

Caution: Whatever items you use, they tend to experiment putting things in their mouth like a toddler so make sure items are safe for them in all scenarios.

While getting dressed, she would place the garment flat on the bed so she could see the tag and that's how her clothes would end up on herself backwards. I would somehow change things out with her before leaving for work and make sure she was properly dressed. I must admit that I found myself shortly after that time wearing a blouse inside out and then went the entire day as such. No one even brought it to my attention! I'm not sure if no one noticed; no one cared; or no one had the heart to tell me. HA! I shared it with her that same afternoon and we both had a good laugh about that. We chose the brighter side of life through laughter and looked for anything to laugh about and whereas most days, I've learned to laugh at myself over the years.

> I was startled to find her one afternoon however, sitting on the sofa, wrapped with a blanket around her legs without wearing any pants.

I'm not sure what happened that day; perhaps she couldn't make it to the bathroom in time and then could not find another pair of pants. I only said, "here mom, let's get some clean clothes on before the guys come home." She didn't think a thing of it. The innocence of her mind was being revealed more and more each passing day.

Through the countless stages, there was a period when mom became so engrossed with people on TV that she would wave and respond to their emotions. I accepted her acts of kindness toward them because my mother was such a kind person, and it was just not that important to overcorrect her at times. She asked me once if we needed to send a baby gift to one of the television anchors that was expecting a baby to which I replied, "I'm not sure when her baby is due." That satisfied her.

Before Alzheimer's took deep root and when she was able to stay by herself during the day while I worked, I always left the television on a lighthearted network channel since she had difficulty with the remote. But she figured out how to change it to the national news which remained "on" throughout her day. In fact, I came home one day, and she was quite upset to the point I had to decompress her from the news story she had been watching. She had even called a few family members about that particular news story too. We all know that media shares repeated headlines, and it was easier for her to engage directly with the television people; they never backtalked! She became so frustrated when trying to describe one of the stories but could not remember any details. I promised her that we would watch the news together that evening. I can still picture her in my mind while she sat in the living room, holding her cup of coffee while smiling at the TV. It made me much more aware that as we age, we become oblivious about what is being said in the context of our words. Sadly, it's just sound to our ears. We don't engage as much in the actual content of the conversation.

> They respond much deeper to acts of emotion. I suppose because they, themselves, have lost total control of their own emotion.

Sammy and I hugged goodbye once in front of her and she began to cry as if she were the one leaving. Perhaps her insight was keen enough to understand. Mom would react if someone were smiling on TV regardless of what was being said and likewise with sadness. Her compassion ran deep, so she would be quick to respond with her own emotions, even into the final stages of the disease. Her doctor kept expressing how pleasant she was and that this disease had a way of pealing back our personality traits; eventually revealing the genuine soul of that person. What a compliment she gave in sharing that. True, Alzheimer's robs a person of many things, but it can never truly take our soul, only expose it to who we genuinely are.

I noticed an increasing desire for her sleep, and she would literally fall asleep within a minute. At bedtime, I would pull down the sheets ready to get into bed and glance over to see her pull them right back up as if to dress the bed. In the mornings, I would help her get dressed and change her shoes around because she would put them on the wrong foot. She would spread out a blanket on her sofa chair but couldn't figure out how to get the blanket wrapped around her. The best way to explain would be that her mind acted in reverse function. It explained why she would place her shoes and clothes reversed. She would hang clothes upside down on the hangers. Although I sensed her frustration, I would never mention anything to her.

Navigation Check Point: Durable Medical

You might consider purchasing these items before they are actually needed. That way, you will have them easily available since dementias can bring rapidly change.

- *Walkers. There are many types available. Be alert that the user may not remember that the legs of the walker are not fully stabilized as they sit down or stand up; which will cause them to unexpectedly lose their balance. Hand brakes are also a big stretch for their small hands to grasp. Mom could not even handle hers properly.*
- *Handrails. Pay close attention to bathroom assisted products. Many have suction cup features but between their hand pressure, weight and water, they can be very hazardous if they are not properly secured.*
- *Wheelchairs. If you purchase used items, make certain all screws and bolts are in place with no rips in the support material. Brakes should be verified. Check all sections for wear and tear so it will not give away to weight.*
- *Portable Toilet. I used the portable toilet frame over my stationary toilet until full portable access was needed. It fit perfectly over my toilet and had handrails for access. You obviously need to stay with them at all times in case they lose balance. Always be aware with fall preventions.*
- *Auto Windshield Shades: These worked perfect to block mom's roaming hands and finger to prevent her from opening the car door while we were in motion.*

She began to shuffle her feet instead of taking steps to walk. I'm not sure if it was because she was afraid of losing her balance or from genuine fear with her distorted vision. Since our living environment was small, it likely helped her because large open areas were frightening to her. Furniture, rugs, and tables can also be hazardous.

When she could still carry conversations, she frequently called me mother and sometimes Lee. Much of her memory took her back to her youth but it became increasingly difficult for her to remember those who had already passed. I kept lots of photographs out for her and she would sift through them daily. I tried to keep them on her dresser and I could see where she would move them about. One night, around midnight, I was trying to settle down myself and she brought me a little picture with a smile on her face. She cuddled it in her hands beside her heart and said, "this is Johnny as a baby." That next morning, it was face up on the dresser waiting to be carried around another day. It was her little world and I did everything possible to protect it. When she turned 84, her church family at Philippi Baptist sent her birthday cards. Sammy collected them at the church and delivered them for her birthday. Steve opened each one and read them to her. Oh, how she delighted in them. It took us a while to go through them. I lined the walls and doors with them and kept them up for weeks because she enjoyed them so much.

Jimmy became the name for both Sammy and Johnny. It took me weeks to figure out the reasoning. It was a combination of their names. Of course, our entire family is frequently called by the wrong name. Years ago, mom and I jokingly nicknamed one another Margaret. But when our large family was together and multiple conversations were active, Steve was called Johnny. Jason called Steve. Diane was Debbie. Debbie was Diane and so forth and so forth and most likely for generations to come! We laughed with one another saying, "I'll find out who you are eventually!" Mom frequently referred to our cousins as "the girls" meaning a combination of them all. They live "there" meant different states. She was troubled by a family photo one day because she could not recognize the people by name. She talked about how pretty her mom was in that picture and I replied, "she is just as pretty as my mom." But she didn't understand what I meant so I said, "you are my mom and I think you are beautiful too." She bowed over and began to cry. I asked why she crying and she questioned…

| …"am I your mother?" |

I said, "yes and you are beautiful"! But I can understand the tears. Most women would cry too if they were my mother (trying to make her laugh) *even though there is most likely truth in that statement.*

Mom went to a church function with me one evening and before we left, she said, "I want to talk to that little lady over there; she looks so sweet." As I glanced around, I realized she was talking about herself because she was staring across the room into a mirror, catching her own reflection. I gave her a hug and said, "that little lady IS a sweet lady! That is, YOU!"

My heart was suddenly overcast with clouds that produced tears of precipitation like rain.

Speaking of tears like rain, there was a period when mom would have crying episodes for no reason. It about drove us all crazy. Sammy asked her one day why she was even crying and she said,

> "I don't know who I am."

How do you find *any* words in response to that?

Heart.

Wrenching.

We discovered when we were in the car, she would ride for miles and enjoy the scenery. Quiet as a mouse. Happy as a lark.... which made us happy too. Many times, we would just go for a ride to distract her attention from crying. Johnny would drive us through the mountains which gave us all a break. She had quite a fetish for rocks and everywhere we went, she wanted to stop to get one. Her dad and mom had a passion for earth and nature which reflected in the home papaw had built. He used slate rock to surround their entire home including three large sections of slate stone steps that led up to the house. So, we've always loved rocks. One time on our trips, Johnny stopped at a waterfall area and picked up a smooth pebble for her. She carried that rock in her back pocket and her purse every day for weeks. Who would have thought a small pebble would make such an impact.

Along with her new personality quirks, I kept her well stocked with tissues and lipstick. She loved them both. As usual, I watched her pull tissues out of the box and refold them and place them in her purse, pockets, and dresser drawers. I had to be watchful for the lipstick lids though. I would find them laying lose and that meant a tube of lipstick was somewhere without its lid. Her favorite comb was frequently found in her Bible. She would carry her comb around and I could hear her stroke the spokes like strumming a guitar. It made perfect sense to me though since most of her life, she was a hair instructor and always had a comb in her hand.

She received a gift of cash at Christmas one year and kept it stashed in a few different places. I had already learned her little hiding spots, but this particular time caught me off guard because she brought me her tube of lipstick and needed help digging out the cash she had tucked inside the tube. I've never seen "Benjamin" with such rosy cheeks before!

Public Media Post
December 16, 2019

Love looks beyond circumstance! One of my favorite Christmas events is to attend the Tennessee Theatre for the community holiday movie. Who doesn't love *Wonderful Life*... right? It's a time that I get to spend with my family and I cherish them!

The waiting lines were wrapped around the city block and the theatre was at capacity. We made it in and enjoyed the music and history about the movie being told. The movie began and held mom's attention for awhile but I ended up needing to move because of her chatter. I'm never embarrassed by that but certainly respecting those around us....I moved us over to a dark corner and just stood behind her. That didn't work either. She began to cry (more of an emotion...not actually tears)...and I knew we would need to leave. So, we did. Most would think how disappointing...too much trouble for nothing.

Oh no! Wrong!

> The brief moment that we had already shared with family was absorbed and until next year...we will meet there again. I'm not upset that we had to leave, mom was fine...just the chatter that immediately stopped once we were in the car. You see, it really IS a wonderful life. And we have to soak up all of this life we can. It doesn't stop me from taking mom out. She actually thrives on people. Don't let circumstances steal your joy. We all know where that comes from! Real joy comes from the Lord. And His love reaches way beyond our circumstances. So forever let His praises ring!
>
> Love looks beyond circumstance!

I'm not sure if it was due to her inability to hear the water run or her vision with seeing the faucet properly but, on several occasions, I would come home to find the water running full force. I had to tell the guys as they came through the house at any time, to glance over the sinks and make sure the water was off. One afternoon, I noticed the water hose in the back yard running full force. She had watered the garden flowers and I could tell it had been flowing for quite a long time because I had a small river. I was so frustrated but fought back my rage of comments like...why...what were you thinking...could you NOT see or hear the water running? Man, it's hard when you're in those moments to hold the attack of a tongue.

> Remember Donna! The water is insignificant. Certainly, it's insignificant to what is really occurring in their mind.

Mom had a television show that she loved to watch about a family with quintuplets. She loved to watch the babies. The word baby became a complete conversation about a thousand times every day.

The babies.

The babies. The babies. The babies!

On and on and on…all day long; the babies!

We tried the pacification of bringing her a baby doll to hold. She looked at it and said, "how pretty" but then held it by its foot without care. We figured she had raised enough babies herself and recognized she did not want to care for any others! I actually got a laugh out of that.

During moments of unsettled behavior, you try everything to occupy their time and most days you find yourself looking for anything to "pacify" them but the attention span grows shorter and shorter like the flight of a gnat. I don't say that to be disrespectful but rather, descriptive about behavior. Music calmed her. Holding her hand calmed her.

She preferred small areas rather than large rooms with a lot of people. In fact, regarding the repetitive word baby, I believe she saw herself as a baby. She understood we were taking care of our baby.

Repetitive phrases (and I mean ALL DAY LONG) included "I want to go to church;" "I don't know where it is;" "Donna;" "Donna;" "Donna."

My name, Donna had multiple meanings to her. Over the course of the disease, words became fewer and fewer. But then, occasionally we would hear her say a small sentence. Sometimes, her repetitive phrases would be like air seeping out of a balloon. One constant release of jumbled words and then one large inhale of air. Words rush out; one large inhale.

She would rock her body back and forth at the same time in a conversation with herself and this action would even occasionally cause her asthma to flare because of the forceful talking and constant activity.

> We always watched for the full moons because it never failed, her behavior would be non-stop for a full 24 hours.

I was not very nice during those sleepless nights. I am a bear without some sort of sleep but would describe those nights as life with an infant, you sleep when you can and where you can. I understand how sundowners can occur with patients. If you're not familiar with that term, it can be its own storm. They basically sleep all day and are up all night. They become increasingly active during the night. Even though you yearn for peace and quiet during the day, you learn NOT to tip-toe around them like a baby because believe me, you need your sleep at night.

Public Media Post
January 2, 2019

This solemn look. 2019. NYD. During the evening, I positioned mom facing me to help keep her alert. She has slept most of the day. NYEve she talked until around 1:00 a.m. then on NYD I had difficulty just keeping her awake. She does that occasionally. She finally "woke up" late evening. But this stare. She has been just looking at me. Like a new parent gazes into their newborn's eyes. No words are really needed. The stare is beyond words really. It's like our souls picked up at life's first glance and imprinted for eternity. I wonder what she sees.

Is it sadness in letting go?
Because it is for me.

Is it gratefulness for our lifetime together?
Because it is for me.

Is it gratitude for our relationship?
Because it is for me.

An occasional blink and slight smile to acknowledge my words of "I love you" is enough to fill our hearts for now.

Help me Lord and forgive my selfish heart and desires of this world. I trust Your timing with mom. It will break my heart when You call her home but I thank you for Your immeasurable compassion and mercy over her. Thank you for allowing her to be my earthly mom because she is the one that led me to You.

I am eternally grateful.

I had normal household responsibilities to manage like everyone else but when you are a caregiver, normal responsibilities may not be managed so easily. Particularly when I needed to do something in another room or even mow the lawn. I remember seating mom in front of my large window and secured her into a chair so I could keep my eyes on her while I RAN the mower as fast as I could, not even paying attention to the grass because I could not take my eyes off of her for fear of something happening. I also wondered just what my neighbors thought. She could see me too and would scream my name while crying uncontrollably. I know what you're thinking…have someone else mow my grass or don't mow. Right or wrong, I continued to manage my own responsibilities. I will never forget the look of fear in her eyes and in her voice. It's not just the lawn, I could step down the hallway to place laundry together and she would behave in the same manner. I had to remind myself that I was her security and that remained the reasoning to a lot of her uncontrollable insecurities.

It's hard to refrain from asking them questions of their past but better to just meet them where they are in the moment. Refrain from, "remember the time we went…"

You can never say I love you enough and hearing a response in return but once when she replied "I like you" was very special to me. Almost better than *I love you*. I know we say "I love you" a lot. We find ourselves saying it more as if we long for one more "I love you" to ring through our ears as if it could be the last time we hear it. And, it may be the last time we hear it.

I imagined different scenarios such as her falling, sudden stroke, cancer or her just drifting asleep into eternity. But we can never really be prepared, can we? During Alzheimer's, the person they once were slowly fades away. I feared saying goodbye twice yet that is exactly what happens in this disease.

> You must let them go with who they once were and get to know this new person with acceptance.

It's very frustrating for everyone. You raise your voice with them so they can hear (if their hearing is impaired) and even more so to just gain their attention.

Her small words had big meaning. Her babble had deeper meaning. She would babble and then stop to look at me with a stare as if to question me that I understood her. A moment would pass, and she would begin body rocking with babble again. Even into the bed-ridden stage when she hardly moved, she would still move her mouth with whispers that you could barely recognize. But again, Jesus knew every whisper she ever made in her life and knew exactly what her heart was saying. Just as He knows our thoughts and heart. You can never escape His love.

Increasingly over time, she had mild body jerks in her arm and shoulders at random. I believe it was just loss of muscle control because it wasn't like a seizure movement, just exaggerated twitches from time to time. The entire body slowly loses control. I emphasize the word slowly. Even at the end of life because even in death, it's all very surreal.

If you magnified a tiny grain of sand, you would see amazing things in its texture and content. Once a boulter or piece of earth crust, over thousands of years, repeated erosion ground it into dust over time. Broken down, by the powerful pounding of the waves, churning over and over through time. We certainly can't compare the time scale of a grain of sand to that of dementia, but you get the idea of the slow progression with the breakdown of this disease.

Even though everything in her physical body failed, she still had comprehension of music and church right up until about a year and half before we lost her. She repeatedly said, "I want to go to church, I want to go to church, I want to go to church." I did everything I could to make that happen and I'm not sure who gained more from going to church…mom…or me. It wasn't easy getting there either. You know what I mean. With or without her, there are always Sunday morning conflicts and darts that come from no one other than the devil. He knows what blessing or encouragement you are going to receive in going to church so he certainly doesn't want you to benefit from that. I remember when my children were babies, the struggles we had to just get us to church would be exhausting. Physically and mentally. One particular Sunday, there we sat, in the balcony, top row, middle of the pew…and I just silently and inwardly cried. You might say a release but for me, I was just crying out to my Father in my own babble. He knows everything on our heart so why not just cry out to Him, even in babble. And He knew mom's babble and exactly what it meant. Going to church doesn't grant you salvation. But, it surrounds you and lifts you with His people that give you strength….His strength and encouragement to face another day.

Taking mom to church, or anywhere for that matter demanded physical strength and extra time. With or without a wheelchair, if you think about a toddler, add at least 100 lbs.; only a toddler will walk with you and want to do so independently. An elder just wants you to be there with them. The strength it takes to walk with them is physically demanding on both of you. When toddlers are emotional, they can be soothed. There is no pacifying an elder. Crying and chanting will continue. My neighbors likely thought abuse because of my loud voice but it was because I was fighting to get her attention. When I brushed her teeth, she would bite the toothbrush. I'm positive there were sensitive things going on but if I could get her teeth in the morning and night, I was doing good. Mouthwash had to stop because she would swallow it but then spit out the toothpaste in the floor. I just did the best I could with dental. I mistakenly used a dishwashing liquid as toothpaste for myself one evening and didn't realize it until I had it in my mouth! Hopefully, I did not use that with her. It could have been why she would spit things out!

| So…spitting. Yes, there is spitting. |

If you give them something to eat and they don't want it in their mouth…out it comes.

During our Christmas Eve Candlelight Service one year, I closely watched her for fear she would spit out the tab of bread during observance of the Lord's Supper and land in the back of someone's head in front of us. We'd also been fortunate that she normally swallowed her caplets and medications. There had been periods when she would spit them across the room, and I would have to quickly chase them down before the pets found them. Animals hear that little ping sound when anything hits the floor and they come running.

There could have been issues with taste or texture too. Mom would clinch her mouth closed if she wanted no part of either medications or eating. I tried using a bib for a few weeks but even that became a hassle. I just made sure we had excessive napkins close at hand.

It didn't take long for me to realize I could NOT leave her alone in a vehicle for any period of time. There were a few instances when I knew I could get in and out of a small stop quickly and while keeping a visual on her, but I could see her crying and it was just too stressful on her apart from the fact someone could report her to the police. I surely did not want to explain THAT! And then she began calling out to others quite loud yelling, "hey, come here."

She would actually grab ahold of people too while in public. She would hold their hand and kiss them and tell them she loved them. I didn't find it embarrassing but in today's world, you just can't do that. She never wanted me out of her sight during those months. I really had to keep an eye on her while I was driving in the car too because her roaming hands would eventually tug on the car door handle. I mean, her hands just never stopped moving around. She would roll the window down and not bat an eye in the wind. I ended up purchasing a vehicle dash shade and I placed it in between her car seat and the door. That essentially hid the car handle from her roaming hands. It's amazing what simple things you come up with during the multiple transitions of their actions and personality changes.

Naturally as we age, there are physical and mental changes that occur with everyone regardless of a dementia on the horizon.

Circumstances can also change our direction as we travel this journey called life. We must adjust the sails according to the winds of change. The journey may be long. It may be a rough voyage. But everyone must sail their own course and if your journey includes the role as a caregiver, let me encourage you to continue to love them through the journey because they, along with the course itself, will most definitely change.

Diligently support them in whatever way possible. Beneath their oddities, they still exist.

They've just been submerged a bit deeper into an abyss of something beyond anyone's control and they need your steady hand to help navigate. Their grip will soon slip away, but you might find comfort in holding their hand along with the approaching winds of change.

Mom's Journey

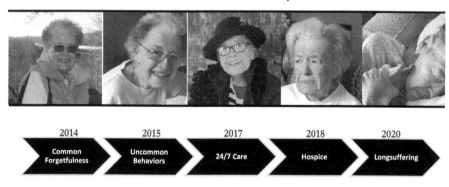

Isaiah 40:8

The grass withereth, the flower fadeth, but the word of our God shall stand for ever.

Chapter Six

Beauty Within

Beauty is in the eyes of the beholder, right? Being artistic in any nature, the artist "feels" their work. Whether it is expression in a poem, painting, singing, or anything else with artistic illustrations, the artist dips deep into their soul. That is where genuine beauty dwells. There is nothing pretty at all about Alzheimer's. The progression peels away layer after layer of a person's life until the soul is all that remains. The caregiver looks beyond the ugliness of destruction. There have been waves and waves of mom's progression. She would plateau for stages and then dive. Those dives could be short stages or be brief. It is constant change though and there is a brief new normal every day.

You ask where you may find the beauty within at this point. It is in the eyes. It is in the innocence. It is within the hands that clinch tightly to anything within the grip. It lies within a faint smile as if to say, "thank you." Thank you for loving me through this ugliness.

Mom lost the ability to speak but made the sweetest little clicking sound with her tongue. The last I heard her say, "I love you" was on February 28, 2020. Why do I know? Because you want to remember those moments like a baby taking their first step.

> Our bodies grow old and regardless, if you experience Alzheimer's or just age with time, our bodies simply wear out.

What lies beneath the surface is who we are. I know; our culture, life experiences, education, family rearing and all other experiences attribute to who we become but it is all really a choice too. When your roots are deep, you can withstand storms. Look at the daisy that pokes its face through a crack in a concrete sidewalk and still blooms. It is the beauty within us. It is perseverance against the odds.

I typically hit the ground running on most days, but I soon reached a point myself like I was just hitting the ground. I remember most days before waking up, I would lay in bed and try to build up my own strength even before rolling out of bed because I knew the physical toll it would take with just getting mom dressed while mixed with an equal dose of my own mental strains. Still, I always made sure she was sporting something cute. Their types of clothing will change because their body flexibility is a major ordeal. They cannot flex and bend, so I began dressing her in sweatshirt style tops and sweaters. No buttons. No zippers. Definitely pull-up pants. Mom never liked gowns, so I kept her in lose denim until she became too frail to move. Before she was totally confined to the bed, I would be so out of breath many times just bending down for long periods of time to get her feet through the pant leg. They can't point their toe and steer their foot into the pant leg, so their foot goes flat-footed down the pantleg as you dress them. I dressed mom in loose jeans mostly because they were easy to wear and clean. There will definitely be (MANY) soiled garments and you should be prepared how to manage the garment clean-up.

It. Gets. Nasty!

If you have a child, do you focus on the memories from the clean-up ugliness in their infant days? Of course not. Those memories don't linger because your acts of love extend beyond the mess. Your love is a reflection from beauty within.

Some of the major dives mom experienced were typically the result from her frequent UTIs. I never realized the affects that a UTI has on a senior adult. We tried very hard to keep mom drinking as much water as possible, which also meant more bathroom trips. It became a vicious cycle. Mom would drink the flavored waters but didn't like regular water very much. When she began to slip away, she refused to open her mouth for food and drinks. I tried many times to pry her mouth open with a spoon to feed her. I knew she was hungry, but she would simply refuse. In her later days, I used a straw to hold small portions of water and released it in the side of her mouth.

Public Media Post
December 3, 2018

"The Grey Roses of Alzheimer's"

A glimpse of my personal notes as we walk this path. It is harsh but real. Every day is different. There is no rhyme or reason to it. Perhaps it will provide some encouragement to others. Yesterday, we had to prop you up in the large wheelchair and use a pillow to pad around you with a seat belt because you did not want to sit up. It seems mean but it helped keep you upright. The leaning is so prominent at times and it seems like the muscles are trying to contract to the point of a fetal position. Every muscle seems flinched and fighting.

Is it fighting for life?

Fighting with fear?

Fighting to communicate?

I'm not sure; but we are fighting for you too.

You have become so frail, and I worry that I may hurt you in just positioning you. I'm afraid we have reached the point to use this wheelchair most of the time now. Most of your words are babble. You sometimes stare right through me. You sometimes stare into the distance. I pray it is a glimpse of heaven that you see but I know if it were heaven in your sight...you would surely collapse with the shear desire to go. I selfishly still want you here though. I'm not sure how I will carry on without you. I fear to even think of losing you even though I know realistically time is short. I praise God for allowing you to be with us for your 87 beautiful years thus far. You are simply beautiful to me even in this end stage. I miss who you were. I miss who you've become in this awful disease because of your innocence. Alzheimer's is a cancer.

> It takes its toll on everyone. I'm not sure who hurts worse...you...or your family walking the journey beside you that love you beyond words.
>
> We ourselves, are babbling.
>
> One thing I know, it is hard, but we will continue to walk with you to the edge of this earth together and until you take the Lord's hand home.

I watched over her as she slept curled in an infant position in this last stage. It is shocking to see the frailty of someone's life at journey's end. Drastic weight loss, aspiration, wheezing, eyes closed at all times, sleeping 24/7 and skin discolorations. There were days that pockets of swelling would occur. I suppose from poor circulation. Her eyes and temple areas became hollow and sunken. It seemed contradictive too, but I was so amazed at the strength of her will to live. With frequent pressure ulcers near the end, it's as looking eye to eye of this ugly monster. Deep seeded in the bones. Lying in wait for an opportune time to surface. Almost like looking into the face of a demon. This disease is a demon.

> I've often wondered, was this Satan's last stab at torment to mom's precious soul?

He knew that mom's soul belonged to Jesus and she forever belonged in His hands. Thankfully, mom was unaware of the spiritual battle that surrounded her. She would be completely healed soon and once her spirit left her body here on earth, her eyes would immediately see Jesus. What an awakening! Chains forever gone and her body completely transformed into a new and eternal perfect health. Forever. Can you just imagine? That's what it will be for Believers in Christ. I found myself jealous of mom's new beginning.

Oh, I will be there too when He calls me home. What a glorious day that will be when we are all called home. That, my friend, is genuine and eternal beauty within.

Notably for mom during her battles, UTIs were an underlying culprit that developed quickly. After a point and even after a two-week span of antibiotics, they kept her on a low dose to further curb infection all the while, we understood this is nowhere near a cure for UTIs. It continued in cycles and then one particular day, her body just stopped producing urine. She kept a very unpleasant look about her which I'm sure was indication of pain, yet she never moaned. With her history of UTIs, it was obvious even after the round of antibiotics, her kidneys began to fail. Her lack of being able to produce led to placement of a catheter. I asked the nurse if this was permanent which her one-word reply: "yes." Even still, you can't gage a catheter placement as approaching death. Remember, our bodies are all different. At that point, we still fully dressed her and kept her in the wheelchair during the day. It was a different routine for certain and I found it to be a bit scary because I knew things were immediately changing. I was able to adjust in monitoring her fluids and proper handling while ironically (and at the same time), the world was in its own crisis with COVID-19 (C-19). I was blessed to be working from home during this phase. Another hidden blessing to give me extra and final time with her.

Navigation Check Point: Diet

If you are transitioning a loved one in these circumstances, consider the following:

- *Diabetes. With diabetes, there are areas of concern with regard to diet. As long as mom could tolerate eating and chewing, we offered as much meat protein as possible. Try to keep a good balance between greens and their digestion system which definitely changes.*
- *Tastebuds. Appetite will likely change. They forget to eat and what is offered to them may bring a frown because of the change in their tastebuds.*
- *Chewing. They may chew a long time with hardly anything in their mouth signaling they have forgotten how to swallow. Certainly, notify your nursing team with your options moving forward.*

- *Meats*. Fish is a great source of protein and easiest of meats for them to chew. Mom was allergic to fish and we opted for other meat options but the meal must be tender and offered in small bites.
- *Drinks*. It becomes difficult for them to drink from a regular glass. The only adult type of sippy top I could find was in a water bottle found at convenience stores with a snap top similar to a sippy bottle. It worked for us and I stocked up on them when I found them and recycled the lids for times I could not find the same product.

It became obvious that mom didn't want to be moved within another week's time. Putting her back in bed one evening, I noticed some black spots on her backside. The next morning, it was much worse. By the time Hospice came on their normal visit, it had blistered into a very ugly site. I was shocked at the fast rate it had developed. The nurses were not taken by surprise though.

> Once the body begins to die, it all begins to shut down.

I remembered the ulcer experience from months earlier when we battled a foot ulcer and had to do 20-minute foot baths every day. Sure, squeeze that into your other daily responsibilities and keep the pets away from the swirling water. Again, things like that are easier said than done.

I will add that her socks began to swell her ankles, so I had to change them over to a loose fit style; a little more difficult to find. Amid the changing routines, mom would spend her remaining days basically asleep even through bathing and rotating her bed positioning. While still attempting to feed her, I had one baby spoon in my kitchen from when my children were little and used it to scoop out food particles that she wouldn't swallow. It's not like she could hold her mouth open for me to do that either, I would just try to softly move the spoon around in her mouth. I worried a lot about the condition of her teeth and too much poking around her mouth could dislodge a tooth or even her bridge at that point. Soft foods were her only diet but there were things that she would chew two times and then drift back to sleep with the food remaining in her mouth. Soft eggs, mashed potatoes, baby food varieties, puddings, mashed beans, bananas with dabs of smooth peanut butter or any other very soft foods were the only items she could do. She continued to slowly wither away in her body mass. In fact, her calf muscles just seemed to disappear as did all of her limb muscles.

She aspirated one morning and that was extremely difficult to watch. I wasn't sure she would make it again through this episode. We were both so helpless. She had begun to lose the ability to swallow. She became drawn into a fetal position most of the time and yet her strength remained. She was so tightly bound now. A few times, the nurse was not able to get a blood pressure reading because her arm was so tightly bent and locked into position. It was rare to see her eyes during this phase but when they opened, they were very glossy. Sometimes very dark and other times she had tiny pupils. Her skin tone drastically changed, and it was obvious many changes were taking place. Lack of blood flow, shallow breathing, and erratic breathing.

Several people would approach me in different conversations, and I quickly identified with their fear. I've seen it before in my own eyes. When another one would confide in me, I saw them seeking words of encouragement because they had just entered the sinking world through receiving a loved one's diagnosis. It's a look as if to say aloud even without words of, *please prevent this from happening; remove me from this unknown world; tell me it's going to be ok*. On, and on, the thoughts rambled like throwing puzzle pieces onto the floor and trying to sort through it all with dignity and assurance.

I thought I noticed a faded smile during one of the last moments her eyes looked into mine. Or maybe she was seeing Heaven's doors open up for her homecoming. I don't know. All I know is that those faded eyes were going to permanently close soon and the minute her spirit left her body here on earth, her eyes would open into the presence of Jesus. I found myself jealous. Eye expressions without speaking words such as, *please take me with you, how will I go on without you, I wish we could have just one more day together*. On, and on, my own thoughts rambled with those puzzle pieces on the floor while searching for grace.

> My own days teetered between depression and restlessness.

I was thankful that I was able to work from home during the C-19 quarantine. It served to keep my emotions focused while working in my home setting. Some weekends though when by myself, the days were very long. I can typically piddle my weekends away but some days, I let things get the best of me with depression. I found myself not even wanting to sit outdoors to watch the birds. I would literally sit and stare. That is such bizarre behavior for me and I hated it. I remembered earlier during this journey and at times, mom would do the same. I wondered increasingly more, just what was in her mind during those moments.

I couldn't even express what was in my own mind. Worlds apart, yet both colliding and changing like the creation of something new. When death is imminent, there is nothing that you can do but wait. Listening to one of my favorite ministers one Sunday, the topic was prayer. In particular, *pray without ceasing*. His sermon mentioned how our prayers can intercede for others and my mind went to mom. She would never want to be laying there in her condition. Is this what the Lord wants? I can't really say that my prayers for mom were, *Lord please take her*. I found myself talking to the Lord in more of a "trusting His plan and timing" conversation.

Navigation Check Point: The Caregiver's Well-Being

- *Time Management. If you are fortunate to have a routine schedule, keep it as much as possible. I was blessed that I could continue working my normal career and then afterwards, change into my caregiving role. It's all very difficult to manage but will help if you can stick to a routine.*
- *Escape. Sometimes, just 10 minutes stepping away offers an escape. Many times after leaving work and on my way home, I would stop at the local library park and just sit for 10-15 minutes of doing absolutely nothing. Escape is mentally necessary for the caregiver though. Walk, bike, drive, hot shower/bath, do what pleases you that provides you with a break.*

- *Diet.* So much focus on your loved one can prevent you from taking care of your own diet. Try to eat a balanced healthy meal so you can continue in your own best of health. It's too easy to eat junk food anytime but don't neglect your own protein.
- *Breaks.* Believe me. Take them when you can. You know what works best for you.
- *Career.* Be honest in communicating with your leadership team and co-workers with what you are facing. If there are opportunities for counseling assistance, it's not a bad idea to tap into that program. Talk, communicate, continue your professional role as long as possible. Having a career can offer your mind a very needed change from what you are facing as a caregiver.
- *Prayer.* Accept as many prayers as people offer you. You will feel them. Never be embarrassed in asking for prayer. Prayer is our major shield and covering.
- *Devotionals.* My minute devotionals were a major thing that got me through every day other than the prayers from my family and friends. Listen to them in the car. Read them before getting out of your car at work. Many times, I would play a recording of The Bible while at home. Just hearing it in the background gave me perfect peace.
- *Sounding off.* Cry when you need to. Those times will come and will never be planned but it is a release of emotion that needs to surface. It's ok. You're not alone.

With her being confined to the bed, I had to get familiar with the new routine of grabbing the pad beneath her because the skin is so very fragile with the slightest tug. One morning after feeding her a bite or two of fruit and oats, I slowly moved her to her right side. Just that slight movement caused her body to quake and shake. I think she had a mini seizure from it. I was afraid to move her anymore that day. Her little legs became sensitive to move too. Day by day, things were moving at a rapid rate. Hospice increased visits (and some visits were done virtually) during the C-19 virus so a great deal of my time was alone with mom. You would think I would be drawn to sit close by her side, but I did not. You would also think I would pay attention to more things around the house, but I did not. Apart from my office work, I found myself in a robotic state of mind. I would occasionally step outside to watch the birds but that was about it. I suppose I had an understanding about it and what this time represented.

Pulling away.

I thought a lot. In my own mental ramblings, I wondered if that's what the Lord wanted for me. Solitude. Depression is the alternate. As I've mentioned earlier, I did struggle with that from time to time. Some days would absolutely drag by. We could no longer go anywhere. This C-19 virus had EVERYONE locked inside their homes too. COVID-19 was just one component about death for me in 2020. I yearned for contact but was forced to withdraw. I concluded that the Lord was my only shelter and comfort between this battle of C-19 and death. I had figured if the C-19 virus ever entered my home, it would for certain take mom but that was never the case. Regardless, I tried to keep my thoughts on higher things while mom continued to slip slowly away.

> Both, being drawn to our Father's arms. Me, figuratively speaking and mom in her own approaching reality with her eternity.

The beauty within may surround us with life's thorns but they do produce such beautiful roses in a Christian's eternity.

I didn't know how much longer mom's body could physically last. It was just unspeakable to watch how every day, she continued to wither and linger.

How. On. This. Earth… was she *still* here?

She became just a skeletal frame of a person. She would NEVER want to be here in this condition. NO ONE would want to remain in this condition. One hidden blessing was that pain never really surfaced. She would have a frown on her face a lot though as a look of discomfort but never any moaning or exclamations of pain. I approached her side one morning (September 12, 2020) and she looked up and with a very faint sound said, "Donn.." Her eyes closed afterwards. That was a golden moment for me. A true beauty within.

Listen. Don't let the devil steal joy from your adversities. You heard me correctly. What the devil intends to destroy, the Lord can use for His higher purpose and glory (Genesis 50:20). If we but a moment, could step back and see things from His perspective, we would gain a whole new attitude about life, challenges, and our struggles. So, when adversity strikes, count it as joy as described in James 1:2-4. It may seem unrealistic but, you will gain a heightened sense of trust in Christ which brings His perfect peace and therefore, produces stronger faith and perseverance. Happiness is temporary, but real joy is a gift from God.

Adversities still continue in life. First, there is "business" with death that must be handled. And, at once. The notifications, the accounts, the burial, the funeral, the wardrobe, the prescriptions, the obituary, the service, the music, the songs, the clean-up of their belongings, all swirling around you.

And then, the silence.

My private writings, which are now public that you are reading, was my outlet. Once I felt led to actually publish this book, my goals were simple with two questions I had asked myself. Does it honor God? And, is it encouraging to others? If the answers were always yes, then I continued to pursue. There were times my words would flow onto these pages like water. Then periods of time would pass like a drought. I would literally not even look at my writings.

But I kept returning to my journal and life continued to flow like a swift current. Being very close to my mother's sisters (my aunts) over our lifetime, I would do anything in caring for each of them. Our family bonds have always been close. During earlier years, our family began to oversee care for Lee which was heart wrenching to watch her fade. I had also been overseeing care for my other aunt, Betty who lived alone whereas I did everything possible to secure and protect her future. Observing mom, and two of her sisters face such distinct obstacles, each being affected very differently and at altered paces is why I know, this journey affects everyone and every family uniquely. Logic is gone. You face every day with a new question mark. We suddenly lost Betty, mom's youngest sister in February 2021. That blind-sided me. I was not prepared to lose her so quickly. Regardless, through life's continued adversities and challenges, staying grounded in my personal devotions guided me to the Lord who always carried me through.

In March 2021, I began editing and reading through these pages again. And do you know what I found? Well, if you are looking for improper writings and possible errors, you've most definitely found them reading over my pages, but it did a newfound thing for me in March. It renewed me with my own writings of encouragement. The very thing that was one of my simple goals. Maybe it's because I feel these words so deeply and have poured my soul onto these pages, but I was encouraged by my own words that day. And I needed that encouragement because of other struggles that I faced. So yes, adversities continue in life. He never said this world would be easy, but He did say He would always be with us. Even until the end.

Mom? She's good. She's much more than good.

Me? I've never seen myself as beautiful or having a beautiful life. I'm pretty messed up in fact. But if He can use these words through my personal journey, then who am I to question His greater plan? He delights bringing beauty from ashes.

I do pray my writings have encouraged your heart but mostly led you to the Captain of my ship. He is the only way I held the strength to endure the depths of adversity while sailing through the multiple oceans of life. Those waters run deep. But His love runs deeper and there is certainly no greater beauty within.

2 Corinthians 5:17

Therefore, if any man be in Christ, he is a new creation; old things are passed away; behold all things are become new.

Chapter Seven

Steady Course

Yea, though I walk through the valley of death, I will fear no evil for Thou are with me. Until you empty yourself to Him, you'll never begin to see His power. My brother Steve once said he believed that Sampson was a scrawny fellow. I asked him why. He said, "because that's how God shows His power...through the impossible." Sampson had strength through his hair, right?

Wrong. Sampson received power through God.

While working from home during C-19, my brothers were limited with some visits. It all worked for the good though and enabled me to spend that extra and very personal time with mom while having the ability to work from home. It was very important for me to obviously continue working; I love my career and the business where I work. It also provided me with my own outlets for projects and professional conversations apart from the dementia days. Working gave me important focus through those extreme days. To be honest, I rarely even listened to the news during that time.

Working from home I closely examined reflections about my life, my family, my friends, my everything. I thought a lot about mom in her younger years while we were children. Four busy children with a single-family income (my dad) until mom began her career. She would take me everywhere with her and there were two hobbies that she enjoyed as her own escape. Sewing and reading. Growing up in a small town may seem boring but to the hometown people, you know where all the treasures exist.

> Mom knew where to find her hidden treasures.

At the local cloth store and at the public library. I hated going to the cloth store to shop for material because there was this horrible smell as you entered the small fabric store. Mom always said it was the chemical dies in the material, but I never liked going there because it would burn my eyes. One of the landmarks in Cleveland was the public library. I liked going there because beyond the large wood entry doors revealed a large spiral staircase. I felt like I was entering an old castle. Inside the doors, the rooms were dimly lit because it was an old house that had been converted into a library. There were a lot of lamps, antique sofas and chairs and rugs. In between the secret passages that were within the home, one could also find another secret passage of escape while reading books. Mom loved a good romance and a little mystery. She let me roam around in that old place. The floors would creak with every step. You had to be quiet too (obviously because it was a library). I had no idea at the time, but mom valued the importance of keeping her personal hobbies active while raising four children. We gave her good reason to want to escape. When my brothers were young, she took them with her downtown to pay a bill and left the boys in the car. She dashed inside (just steps away) and confident that nothing could possibly happen within the short time she would be gone. Keep in mind, these were the years that people were so genuine and trustworthy, so safety was a given in a small town. When she returned to the car however, there was a police officer leaning into the car door window and all of my brothers were crying.

"What in the world has happened, officer? I just stepped inside for a minute!"

The officer replied, "well, I walked by and the boys started screaming that their mom had been hit by a car and was gone."

Goodness gracious, the startled reaction!

I shouldn't overlook the time that a frog was released by one of my brothers into the baptism pool while during a service. Now there's a memory, this little frog swimming and floating along while dad was leading the congregation in a chorus of *Gather at the River*.

I'm no princess either. It seemed I liked doing things on a much more public scale that involved dumping bubbles into the local college water fountain prominently viewed by everyone in the county. I'm more and more thankful the older I become that social media did not exist in my adolescent years.

Oh, my heavens! The imagination we had as kids! So, mom definitely needed ways to keep herself engaged in her own personal activities that she enjoyed apart from child rearing!

As we grew a bit older, mom and dad enrolled us into piano lessons. What a terrifying place THAT was! It was another old building that had a trillion antiques that you had to roam your way through the packed, dark building into the "music chamber." Looking back, the music teacher would have been a little like a "Ms. Peacock," very eccentric. I personally didn't gain much music knowledge during those days because of pure fear of going into that building. Our parents were loaded with talent and I do appreciate their efforts into providing education for us.

I say this all for a couple of reasons. Those days taught me how to deal with idle time. Mom, with her crafts, needlework, sewing and reading. Dad with his music, piano, gardening, and visitation. All traits that were passed along to us. We never lacked for anything to do. If we complained of nothing to do, we were told to find something to do or else it would be another assigned chore.

Keeping a good pace and steady course is important at every stage in life. Regardless that mom's mind had long passed, her body was still very present, and I needed to maintain my own hobbies and things I cared about beyond her. That's very OK for us to do but it's also very hard to maintain during the difficult dementia days and responsibilities. During some of my depression points while the nation was on the C-19 lock-down, we were introduced to another behavior modification called "social distancing." It was early spring and that meant rain and more rain. There were periods of cold days so, even to get outside for a break was rare. I sometimes just stared into space.

> I felt as if I were waiting on death's door. Almost anticipating an actual knock at the door.

Along this entire journey, my sister-in-law, Diane was such an encourager to me. She continuously sent me text messages, cards, and small tokens to remind me of her prayers for me. I can't tell you how invaluable that was to me. So many days, when I felt like I had come to the end of my sanity, I would see a note from her. She had been through the same journey with her parents and understood the exhaustion and swirl of emotions that connect with the disease and the extent of what it robs from the person and those around them. Diane is a jewel.

You would think I would use all spare time with sitting beside mom, holding her hand, or talking to her. But I didn't. It was quite depressing to step immediately through my front door and see her hospital bed directly at the front window. I didn't like sitting in the living room at all anymore.

There was a ghost of a person there at all times. I'm certain I had begun to pull away because I was just tired of it all. A typical day in mom's world existed of 23.75 hours of deep sleep. Not comatose. Deep sleep. She had been on a total soft food diet for months (mashed potato consistency) and slept during feedings, bed changes, soiled pads, diapers, and draining catheters.

How long can a body physically endure this torment? It boggled my own mind. This was her life but dictated a direct impact on mine. It is the unmentionable actions and undefined definition of love. You simply run out of yourself for another. You best know how to manage your own sanity during this stage.

When she became fetal position, I had to cut her tops in the back to change her clothing every day. Her night sweats were fierce, and mom never was one to sweat but many mornings, her top would be damp. I didn't over dress her or keep the heat up for her, in fact, I kept the house a bit cool. Her body had literally become locked into a position, and it was painful to move her at all. I had to wipe her down every morning because she was gaining a different odor with everything happening in her body. What had been classified as diabetic dry skin (a totally different dry skin), was now more of a shedding, not pealing but flaky. I kept her as clean as possible, including her ears and between her toes but there was just no way to keep atop the fast production of what I describe as decay. This I know is disgusting to read but it provides you with a vivid picture of what death begins to look and smell like.

October 5, 2020, I had some private time sitting across the room from mom watching her. Seeking some encouragement, I reached for my Bible and the old cliché of….it fell open to…well, the pages fell open to John 14. When reading it to myself, I couldn't get past the second verse. I read 1-6 several times to myself. How fitting that God would show me these verses for comfort. I couldn't go to bed without reading it aloud to her. Rather soft in her ears, I read them again.

I could actually see movement in her eyelids in response. I don't know, maybe she heard the voice of Jesus actually speaking to her instead of my own voice.

I kissed her on the forehead and said, "He's preparing you a place, mom. Jesus is preparing your place."

Public Media Post
May 29, 2019

"Hand to Hand"

It's ok to take His hand
When He calls your name.
I know you're just a little scared-
With me it's quite the same.

We've said goodbye so many times;
But this one stops my heart.
It skips a beat then you'll be gone,
I'm really torn apart.

Greater still, assurance calm;
Is deep within my soul.
He stands between us all the while,
Until He calls you home.

So, it's ok to leave this world-
When He calls your name.
There is no greater place to go,
Than with Him from whence He came.

Afterwards you'll greet me too,
When He takes my hand.
All the while, we're not alone-
With Him is where we stand.

And then our days will just begin;
No need to leave that shore.
For eternity we'll share with Him-
And live forevermore!

-Written by Donna Mowery 5/29/19

I could never find myself actually asking the Lord to take her except for one time. Her body could not have weighed more than 60 pounds and in the appearance, seemed almost mummified. This beast took every ounce of her being and stripped every fiber of her life. It was gruesome to watch day by day. Each morning, I would get up expecting her to have passed but would find her still there. Then, on October 24, 2020, I got up, met Sammy and Johnny (who had stayed up all night during that stage) and I had no words. I simply broke. I lost it and began to openly weep; not cry….WEEP. I remember saying aloud, "I can't take it anymore! I can't stand to see her in this horrific condition anymore!" My brothers had no words in response. They had never seen me in this condition either, but it was true. I had reached my own limit. We prayed there together and within the prayer asked that the Lord take her that day. Steve came in later that afternoon and was the one to discover when she had passed softly and quietly while we were in other areas of the house. Being the *"Martha"* that I am, was standing in the kitchen. I believe the Holy Spirit pulled Steve up at the exact moment her spirit left because he went over to check on her and softly said,

| "Guys, she's gone." |

Then, in the blink of an eye, her real life began. She was made purely whole. Perfectly well and walking alongside Jesus. It was Jesus that had walked alongside her all of her years and literally cradled her through the past three years. Like the footprints in the sand where two people are walking and then suddenly one set of footprints disappear. That's when He carries us. He never left her and no doubt in my mind was the first to welcome her home. "Well done, my good and faithful servant."

It was Steve's suggestion for us to pray in thanks to our Father for her life. So, we gathered over her ghost of a body and prayed together again. I had no words to speak in prayer, but I gleaned every word that came pouring out from my brothers. I can't say that my initial reaction was tears. I had cried them all out within the past few years in repeatedly saying goodbye to her. She had already been gone.

> You say "goodbye" to Alzheimer's patients multiple times before they reach their actual passing.

Now, there were immediate calls to make. Arrangements to call to action.

I think what I miss about her the most though is our friendship.

There are moments when for a split second, I think she is still here.

Shortly after losing her, I was sitting outside enjoying the late autumn evening and watching my birds find their nesting spot for the night. There were about 5 bluebirds that flew onto a pine branch above my head. They were chirping and hopping around in the needles. Then, as if an instructor called them to order, they lined up; side-by-side with not a glimmer of light between them. Then stillness fell. That was such a sweet sight and for a split second, I had to catch myself from calling out to mom. She would have adored that sight. We would have sat together side by side, just like the birds and watched. Oh, the simple blessings we miss if we don't watch for them. I miss sharing these moments with mom but I know she is seeing another sight that she longs to share with me…

> …the sights of Jesus in heaven.

It poured rain at her service and the day of graveside. Very symbolic of what was taking place in my heart. And then on that muddy bank, while we huddled beneath the tent together as a family, I said a temporary earthly goodbye to my very best friend. Alice Hooker Southerland.

Oh, but it certainly doesn't end at the graveside. At least not for Believers. There's more because the best is yet to come. We will just keep a steady course until our Father calls us home. How do we do that? We keep our eyes on Jesus. We keep reading His Word. It's our roadmap in life. Yes, it's what my mom and dad taught me, but I've learned it to be truth for myself. It's a choice He gives us all so you can decide for yourself.

One month later I was adrift in different waves called approaching holidays but where chaos and demanding routine previously consumed me, I felt that…

> …my life suddenly became a dead calm.

Even during the holidays, I was surrounded by silence and solitude. Empty nest. Still pushing through the constraints of lockdown with C-19, unable to get fully into swing with normal activities. Wondering…will there EVER be a normal again. But, that's part of life. Bending with the winds of change. This, I know that life is CONSTANT change. And sometimes, the winds of change bring a new direction.

There is always hinderance to what we think our plans should be. For instance, I would have a list of things I could see myself wanting to do if only I weren't pinned down by these caregiver responsibilities. However, no longer having the caregiver role in my life, I still have hinderances that seem to surround me. In other words, I wonder if we hold ourselves down and just make excuses to what we think we want or ought to be doing?

And then sometimes I do wonder what people mean when they say, "you need to take care of yourself." Am I not doing something? What does that mean exactly? Does it mean rest? Does it mean I need to do things for myself? Because I do all those things but the moment I sit down, I am called away for something else like the dryer sounding off "hey, I'm ready now."

I recently watched my son carry a load of laundry in one afternoon and the clothes were already folded. He said he wanted to wash them before donating them, which made perfect sense. Only, when he opened the washer, he dumped the entire stack (still folded) into the washer. I didn't waste my time saying anything else. In fact, I thought I might learn something from this behavior. I chuckled to myself because when I transferred them into the dryer, they were still folded.

Again, I merely put them in the dryer and thought if they dried in the folded position...we could be on the brink of a new discovery! HA!

I think we need more of this along our journey. Learning how to accept different methods and embracing the change. Caregivers never have enough time to regenerate themselves though, and in my case, it's me, the single mom, the career girl, the caregiver, and the do-er of everything. Thankfully, I have a personal Caregiver that is Omnipotent and Omnipresent with me. I think caregiving is like washing someone's feet. It's dirty. Not many answer the call. It's smelly and sometimes foul. It's exhausting. Every day. Every night. Thank you, Lord, that You answered the call to wash my dirty feet too. His grace is unlimited and flows freely. Untapped and unending. Rivers of pure grace. The only time that *the water is significant* for He is the Living Water.

Whatever chapter your own life is currently in, I encourage you to press on. I have now entered into an empty nest chapter. And you know what? I'm struggling with it. I transferred from crazy, hectic, overload to silent, solitude and lonely. Are we ever really settled? No, life is constant change. My challenges now are completely different and I'm trying to just embrace the silence. In one single year of my life, I lost my mom, a close aunt, my sons lost their father, and we lost two pets between ranges of 15-18 years (which were family members to us). All within ten months of each other. That is an incredible amount of loss. I don't want sympathy. I still covet prayers from others. ALWAYS. Because life is rotating like the ocean waves.

> I am still standing on that shore looking into the depths of the horizon. Wondering what storm may surface next.

I'm still recovering from the aftermath of this season's storm and almost just as fearful in my new solitude. My own mind screams, "I can't!" But Jesus calmly and assuredly replies, "but my child, with Me, you can!"

I have a few in my life who's loved ones are just entering into the abyss of dementia days. I can hear their thoughts as they share with me in a ramble of words when it all just comes down to two words, "I can't!"

But child, "with Jesus, you can!"

We don't know what storms are brewing.

But I sure know Who controls the wind.

My other advice for you while entering an abyss of dementia?

Let your loved one be as independent as possible and for as long as possible! For themselves and for the respect of them as a person. The last vacation we took mom was to the beach. We weren't sure how she would do traveling or anything else we might encounter but we figured what was there to lose? It was a turning point with using pull-ups in her clothing because of travel and not being able to get to the restrooms "in time." The travel time in the car went well. She was "entertained." There was still chatter but no major problems occurred. When we went into the hotel room, I wheeled her inside so I could begin unpacking. We looked like an army moving in, there was so much to unload. Regardless, I locked her wheels into place and sat her immediately in front of the picture window overlooking the ocean. Her words, "How beautiful!" My brother and I were amazed yet again at her expression and words. That is what made our trip.

Missing mom sure comes in waves, but the sweet reminders of her life help keep me on course. She kept her faith through all of her own journey. That is what has impressed my life so deeply. Her faith. I could honor her all day with stories but the best message I could share genuinely on her behalf would be this:

Don't miss Jesus.

If you don't know Him, now is your time.

> You can't rely on the reflection of someone else's faith to take you to heaven. It's your personal relationship with Christ that counts.

There is no other comfort in dealing with death than to transfer your hope in Christ. One day, I will sit together with mom again and laugh but my life continues now, and I need to live my life fully. I want a happy life!

Since her passing and trying to just keep my eyes on a horizon, her simple words of "how beautiful" have made a lasting impression beyond description because I apply them so differently to life now. She saw things as if for the first time. I think we forget in our day-to-day routine "how beautiful" things are right before our eyes. Moments that may not seem very beautiful at the time but become lasting memories.

You know there are also moments when you look back and laugh. One of those times, my brother Johnny, my sons and I took her to Daytona. It was our first day on the beach and we went for a walk. Dressed for the beach. Looking like it's our first day on the beach. ALBINO. She suddenly became weak and said she needed to sit down. I had her lean up against me and we sat down on the shore. I struggled to get my phone to call Johnny who was walking just ahead of us. He flagged down a lifeguard truck and they were there to assist us in seconds. They hooked her up to an EKG and fluids right there on the shore while the waves rolled in. The ambulance arrived and I climbed into the back with her. Johnny went to get the car to meet us at the hospital.

So, there we were.

Leaving the beach.

In an ambulance.

And in our swimsuits. Driving down the world's most famous beach, watching the waves go by! Not what I had envisioned on our first day at the beach.

I called Justin and Jarod to let them know what had happened and before hanging up, said, "by the way, can you bring us some clothes?" Finally, around 3:00 a.m., mom was released and we headed back to our hotel. Johnny dropped us off at the front entrance.

We were moving very slow of course and no one was around except the dedicated bellhop. He noticed that we were moving like a pack of stampeding snails. After about ten minutes grazing along, he joined us at the elevator and opened the door for us. We got on and just as the doors closed, we made eye contact to say, "we party hard."

So, apart from everything, we loved to laugh and I think to myself over and over just "how beautiful" my life has been with her. It's all in your perspective. It's all up to you whether you want to see the beauty or not.

I do think it's interesting how I've compared my writings to all things ocean. I'm from East Tennessee and have only visited beaches that boarder the Atlantic Ocean. I've even collected bottles of sand from those beaches. Each bottle is enclosed with beautiful memories. On those visits, I have absorbed everything I could around the ocean. I've often said, it's not the location you visit but the journey that takes you there. There's really something wonderful when you see the ocean after driving 500 miles. The feel of the sand. The sounds of the non-stop pounding of the waves. The life that swims beneath us in the waters. The mist from the sprays.

On and on, I could describe what being around the ocean has meant to me. It has been the only mystical thing that I could begin to compare my own journey with Alzheimer's and how I navigated through the water's depth. Many times, I feared I would sink.

My own memories of life and these experiences that I've journaled may surely fade away. I may encounter the ugliness of dementia myself or be told I have cancer one day. I could even die by accident. God gives us all one life. We all have the same amount of time each new day. 24 hours per day. Our days are limited though, and I don't want mine to wash away with the tide. This book in my personal life has come to an end. I'm looking onto a new horizon now wondering in my thoughts, "what's next, God?"

> It may be deep. It may have swells. I'm certain it will hold storms. But this I know. My Father will be there with me.

Not that He needs to prove anything to me, but He has. He has proven His faithfulness to me.

God has given me this day and I don't need to worry about the next. Planning is good. Goals are great. But we shouldn't let the devil steal our joy from the beauty of this day even amid the storms. Keep your eyes on the goal but enjoy the scenery that your journey holds. You might just miss out on something wonderful. After all, there really is sunshine beyond the clouds.

So steady course! And remember, if you hear rumblings of thunder in the distance and your weatherman calls for approaching storms, pull down the patio umbrella, and batten down the hatches mate!

Be assured that beyond those approaching clouds, a rainbow surely exists with God's promise of tomorrow.

And, consequently, it's not really the end.

It's merely an amazing beginning of an eternal voyage

for us Believers.

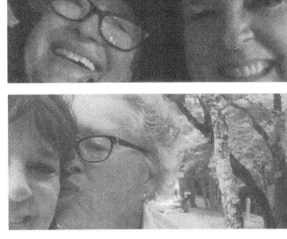
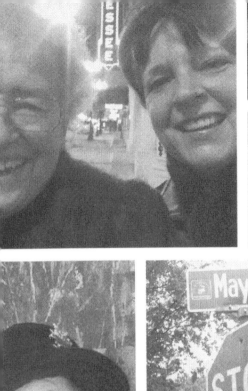
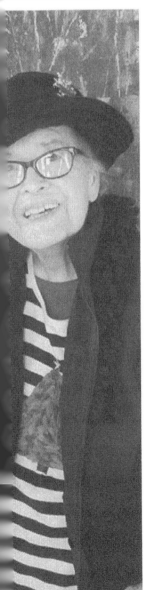
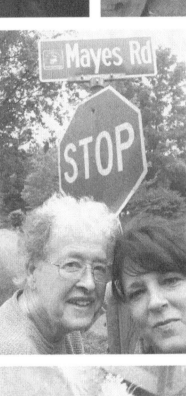
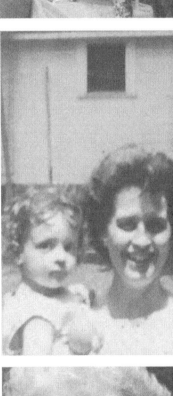
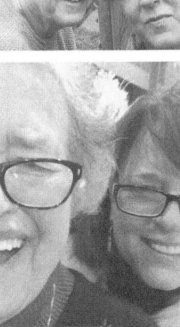
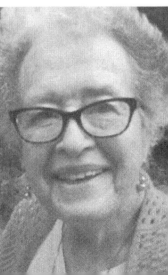

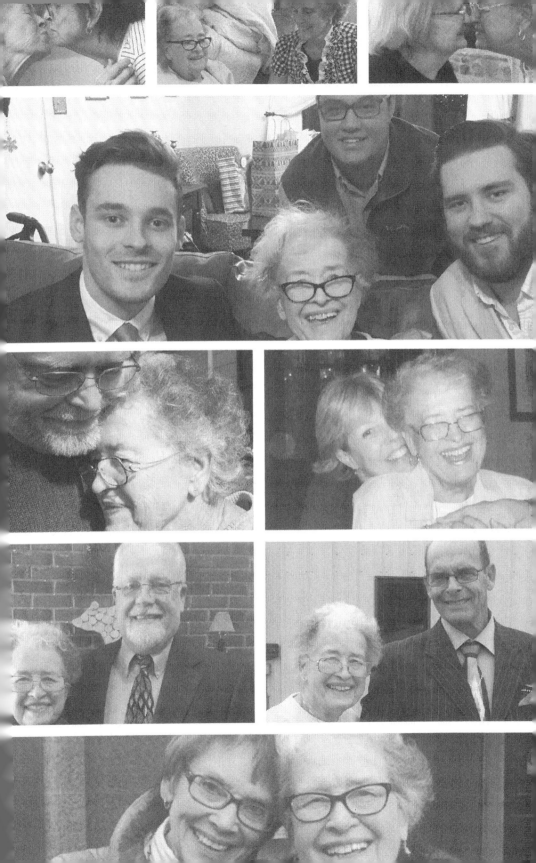

King James Version
Scripture References
Listed in written journal order reference

Inset Cover:

2 Corinthians 4:17-18 ¹⁷For our light affliction, which is but for a moment, worketh for us a far more exceeding *and* eternal weight of glory; ¹⁸while we look not at the things which are seen, but at the things which are not seen: for the things which are seen *are* temporal; but the things which are not seen *are* eternal.

Chapter One:

Lamentations 3:21-24 ²¹This I recall to my mind, Therefore have I hope. ²²*It is of* the LORD's mercies that we are not consumed, Because His compassions fail not. ²³*They are* new every morning: Great *is* thy faithfulness. ²⁴The LORD *is* my portion, saith my soul; Therefore will I hope in Him.

Chapter Two:

Hebrews 6:19 Which hope we have as an anchor of the soul, both sure and stedfast, and which entereth into that within the veil;

James 5:14 Is any sick among you? let him call for the elders of the church; and let them pray over him, anointing him with oil in the name of the Lord:

Chapter Three:

Psalm 61:2 From the end of the earth will I cry unto thee, when my heart is overwhelmed: lead me to the rock that is higher than I.

Job 1:1-19 ¹There was a man in the land of Uz, whose name was Job; and that man was perfect and upright, and one that feared God, and eschewed evil. ² And there were born unto him seven sons and three daughters. ³ His substance also was seven thousand sheep, and three thousand camels, and five hundred yoke of oxen, and five hundred she asses, and a very great household; so that this man was the greatest of all the men of the east. ⁴ And his sons went and feasted in their houses, every one his day; and sent and called for their three sisters to eat and to drink with them. ⁵ And it was so, when the days of their feasting were gone about, that Job sent and sanctified them, and rose up early in the morning, and offered burnt offerings according to the number of them all: for Job said, It may be that my sons have sinned, and cursed God in their hearts. Thus did Job continually.

⁶ Now there was a day when the sons of God came to present themselves before the LORD, and Satan came also among them. ⁷ And the LORD said unto Satan, Whence comest thou? Then Satan answered the LORD, and said, From going to and fro in the earth, and from walking up and down in it. ⁸ And the LORD said unto Satan, Hast thou considered my servant Job, that there is none like him in the earth, a perfect and an upright man, one that feareth God, and escheweth evil? ⁹Then Satan answered the LORD, and said, Doth Job fear God for nought? ¹⁰Hast not thou made an hedge about him, and about his house, and about all that he hath on every side? thou hast blessed the work of his hands, and his substance is increased in the land. ¹¹But put forth thine hand now, and touch all that he hath, and he will curse thee to thy face. ¹²And the LORD said unto Satan, Behold, all that he hath is in thy power; only upon himself put not forth thine hand. So Satan went forth from the presence of the LORD.

¹³And there was a day when his sons and his daughters were eating and drinking wine in their eldest brother's house: ¹⁴And there came a messenger unto Job, and said, The oxen were plowing, and the asses feeding beside them: ¹⁵And the Sabeans fell upon them, and took them away; yea, they have slain the servants with the edge of the sword; and I only am escaped alone to tell thee. ¹⁶While he was yet speaking, there came also another, and said, The fire of God is fallen from heaven, and hath burned up the sheep, and the servants, and consumed them; and I only am escaped alone to tell thee. ¹⁷While he was yet speaking, there came also another, and said, The Chaldeans made out three bands, and fell upon the camels, and have carried them away, yea, and slain the servants with the edge of the sword; and I only am escaped alone to tell thee. ¹⁸While he was yet speaking, there came also another, and said, Thy sons and thy daughters were eating and drinking wine in their eldest brother's house: ¹⁹And,

behold, there came a great wind from the wilderness, and smote the four corners of the house, and it fell upon the young men, and they are dead; and I only am escaped alone to tell thee.

Job 2:7; 9 ⁷So went Satan forth from the presence of the LORD, and smote Job with sore boils from the sole of his foot unto his crown.

⁹Then said his wife unto him, Dost thou still retain thine integrity? curse God, and die.

Job 42:12 So the LORD blessed the latter end of Job more than his beginning: for he had fourteen thousand sheep, and six thousand camels, and a thousand yoke of oxen, and a thousand she asses.

Colossians 1:17 And He is before all things, and by Him all things consist.

Psalm 147:3 He healeth the broken in heart, and bindeth up their wounds.

Genesis 3:3-21 ³But of the fruit of the tree which is in the midst of the garden, God hath said, Ye shall not eat of it, neither shall ye touch it, lest ye die. ⁴And the serpent said unto the woman, Ye shall not surely die: ⁵For God doth know that in the day ye eat thereof, then your eyes shall be opened, and ye shall be as gods, knowing good and evil. ⁶And when the woman saw that the tree was good for food, and that it was pleasant to the eyes, and a tree to be desired to make one wise, she took of the fruit thereof, and did eat, and gave also unto her husband with her; and he did eat. ⁷And the eyes of them both were opened, and they knew that they were naked; and they sewed fig leaves together, and made themselves aprons.

⁸And they heard the voice of the LORD God walking in the garden in the cool of the day: and Adam and his wife hid themselves from the presence of the LORD God amongst the trees of the garden. ⁹And the LORD God called unto Adam, and said unto him, Where art thou? ¹⁰And he said, I heard thy voice in the garden, and I was afraid, because I was naked; and I hid myself. ¹¹And he said, Who told thee that thou wast naked? Hast thou eaten of the tree, whereof I commanded thee that thou shouldest not eat? ¹²And the man said, The woman whom thou gavest to be with me, she gave me of the

tree, and I did eat. ¹³And the LORD God said unto the woman, What is this that thou hast done? And the woman said, The serpent beguiled me, and I did eat.

¹⁴And the LORD God said unto the serpent, Because thou hast done this, thou art cursed above all cattle, and above every beast of the field; upon thy belly shalt thou go, and dust shalt thou eat all the days of thy life: ¹⁵And I will put enmity between thee and the woman, and between thy seed and her seed; it shall bruise thy head, and thou shalt bruise his heel. ¹⁶Unto the woman he said, I will greatly multiply thy sorrow and thy conception; in sorrow thou shalt bring forth children; and thy desire shall be to thy husband, and he shall rule over thee. ¹⁷And unto Adam he said, Because thou hast hearkened unto the voice of thy wife, and hast eaten of the tree, of which I commanded thee, saying, Thou shalt not eat of it: cursed is the ground for thy sake; in sorrow shalt thou eat of it all the days of thy life; ¹⁸Thorns also and thistles shall it bring forth to thee; and thou shalt eat the herb of the field; ¹⁹In the sweat of thy face shalt thou eat bread, till thou return unto the ground; for out of it wast thou taken: for dust thou art, and unto dust shalt thou return. ²⁰And Adam called his wife's name Eve; because she was the mother of all living.

²¹Unto Adam also and to his wife did the LORD God make coats of skins, and clothed them.

Romans 6:23 For the wages of sin is death; but the gift of God is eternal life through Jesus Christ our Lord.

Romans 3:23 For all have sinned, and come short of the glory of God;

Ephesians 2:8-9 ⁸For by grace are ye saved through faith; and that not of yourselves: it is the gift of God: ⁹Not of works, lest any man should boast.

John 14:6 Jesus saith unto him, I am the way, the truth, and the life: no man cometh unto the Father, but by me.

1 Peter 3:18 For Christ also hath once suffered for sins, the just for the unjust, that he might bring us to God, being put to death in the flesh, but quickened by the Spirit:

Romans 4:25 Who was delivered for our offences, and was raised again for our justification.

John 1:12 But as many as received him, to them gave he power to become the sons of God, even to them that believe on his name:

Acts 3:19 Repent ye therefore, and be converted, that your sins may be blotted out, when the times of refreshing shall come from the presence of the Lord.

Acts 26:20 But shewed first unto them of Damascus, and at Jerusalem, and throughout all the coasts of Judaea, and then to the Gentiles, that they should repent and turn to God, and do works meet for repentance.

Romans 10:13 For whosoever shall call upon the name of the Lord shall be saved.

Luke 10:20 Notwithstanding in this rejoice not, that the spirits are subject unto you; but rather rejoice, because your names are written in heaven.

Hebrews 6:4-6 [4] For it is impossible for those who were once enlightened, and have tasted of the heavenly gift, and were made partakers of the Holy Ghost, [5] And have tasted the good word of God, and the powers of the world to come,

[6] If they shall fall away, to renew them again unto repentance; seeing they crucify to themselves the Son of God afresh, and put him to an open shame.

Chapter Four:

Romans 8:28 And we know that all things work together for good to them that love God, to them who are the called according to his purpose.

Matthew 11:28-30 [28]Come unto me, all ye that labour and are heavy laden, and I will give you rest. [29]Take my yoke upon you, and learn of me; for I am meek and lowly in heart: and ye shall find rest unto your souls. ³⁰For my yoke is easy, and my burden is light.

John 17:20-21 ²⁰Neither pray I for these alone, but for them also which shall believe on me through their word; ²¹That they all may be one; as thou, Father, art in me, and I in thee, that they also may be one in us: that the world may believe that thou hast sent me.

Chapter Five:

2 Corinthians 12:9 And he said unto me, My grace is sufficient for thee: for my strength is made perfect in weakness. Most gladly therefore will I rather glory in my infirmities, that the power of Christ may rest upon me.

Chapter Six:

Isaiah 40:8 The grass withereth, the flower fadeth: but the word of our God shall stand for ever.

Genesis 50:20 But as for you, ye thought evil against me; but God meant it unto good, to bring to pass, as it is this day, to save much people alive.

James 1:2-4 My brethren, count it all joy when ye fall into divers temptations; ³ Knowing this, that the trying of your faith worketh patience. ⁴ But let patience have her perfect work, that ye may be perfect and entire, wanting nothing.

Chapter Seven:

2 Corinthians 5:17 Therefore if any man be in Christ, he is a new creature: old things are passed away; behold, all things are become new.

Psalm 23:4 Yea, though I walk through the valley of the shadow of death, I will fear no evil: for thou art with me; thy rod and thy staff they comfort me.

Judges 16:28 And Samson called unto the LORD, and said, O Lord God, remember me, I pray thee, and strengthen me, I pray thee, only this once, O God, that I may be at once avenged of the Philistines for my two eyes.

Matthew 5:21 Well done, thou good and faithful servant;

Luke 10:38-42 [38]Now it came to pass, as they went, that he entered into a certain village: and a certain woman named Martha received him into her house. [39] And she had a sister called Mary, which also sat at Jesus' feet, and heard his word. [40] But Martha was cumbered about much serving, and came to him, and said, Lord, dost thou not care that my sister hath left me to serve alone? bid her therefore that she help me. [41] And Jesus answered and said unto her, Martha, Martha, thou art careful and troubled about many things: [42] But one thing is needful: and Mary hath chosen that good part, which shall not be taken away from her.

John 14:1-6 [1]Let not your heart be troubled: ye believe in God, believe also in me. [2]In my Father's house are many mansions: if it were not so, I would have told you. I go to prepare a place for you. [3]And if I go and prepare a place for you, I will come again, and receive you unto myself; that where I am, there ye may be also. [4]And whither I go ye know, and the way ye know. [5]Thomas saith unto him, Lord, we know not whither thou goest; and how can we know the way? [6]Jesus saith unto him, I am the way, the truth, and the life: no man cometh unto the Father, but by me.

About the Author

Donna Mowery is passionate about her love of Christ and communicates it through artistic methods such as writing. She has served as a co-teacher of ten years in a leading support group for women at her church in Knoxville, Tennessee. At the turn of those years, she began full-time guardianship and care for her mother.

Her professional career is in healthcare marketing where she enjoys working and growing through the variety of challenges it brings alongside her co-team.

She is devoted to her two young adult children and is inspired through their lives. Her beloved family has always remained her strong roots.

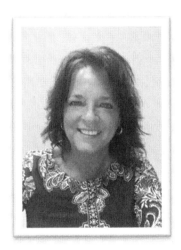

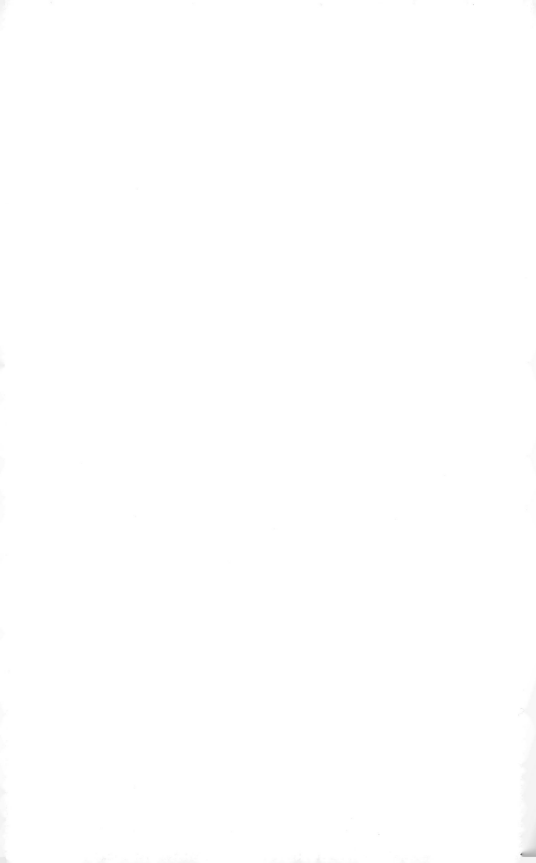

Made in the USA
Las Vegas, NV
06 January 2022